COLLEGE SAFETY 101

COLLEGE

Safety

101

**Miss Independent's Guide to Empowerment,
Confidence, and Staying Safe**

by **KATHLEEN BATY**
The Safety Chick

CHRONICLE BOOKS
SAN FRANCISCO

Copyright © 2011 by Kathleen Baty.

All rights reserved. No part of this book may be reproduced in any form without written permission from the publisher.

Library of Congress Cataloging-in-Publication Data:
Baty, Kathleen.
  College safety 101 / by Kathleen Baty.
    p. cm.
  Includes index.
  ISBN 978-0-8118-6949-2
  1. Universities and colleges--Security measures--United States. 2. Universities and colleges--United States--Safety measures. 3. School violence--United States. I. Title.

  LB2866.B38 2011

  378.1'9782--dc22

2010034905

Manufactured in China

Designed and Illustrated by Candice Leick and Brooke Lunneborg

10 9 8 7 6 5 4 3 2 1

Chronicle Books LLC
680 Second Street
San Francisco, California 94107
www.chroniclebooks.com

DEDICATION

This book is dedicated to four vibrant, loving, and talented young college students, who tragically lost their lives to senseless acts of violence.

Eve Marie Carson, student body president of the University of North Carolina
Lauren Burk, a freshman at Auburn University
Kimberly Smith, a senior at Columbia College, Missouri
Yeardley Love, a senior at University of Virginia

May everyone who reads this book honor their memories by living happy, strong, positive, and empowered lives.

Contents

Introduction:
Meet the Safety Chick

Congratulations, Miss Independent! What an awesome journey. All the hard work of elementary school, junior high, and high school has finally paid off. You are headed to college (or you have arrived already!), getting ready to take the classes and make the grades necessary for becoming the next Nobel Peace Prize winner, CEO of a Fortune 500 company, mother of the year, or even the new host of *American Idol*!

But as you enter this brave new world, it is important to keep your grip on some basic wisdoms. And the one I am concerned with is: You aren't going to get far if you aren't safe!

Personal safety is one of those tricky things we may not think about much consciously until something rears up to remind us—and with safety, that thing can often come with a jolt, sometimes a big one. Sometimes even a big *bad* one. But must it take becoming a crime victim to start caring about your personal safety? The answer of course is, No! My friend Dana Getzinger Foley and I were talking about this the other day. She, like me, was a crime victim in college (you can read her amazing story on page 21), but what she and I continue to commiserate about is the fact that so often people don't actually take the time to educate themselves about or take preventative measures for their personal safety . . . until it is too late.

Here are the facts: The odds of being a victim of a random act of violence are slim to none *if* you make smart personal-safety choices. If you let yourself kind of coast in denial, or general fear makes you avoid thinking about it and educating yourself, your odds of becoming a victim go up. The moment when you head off to college can be intimidating and/or overwhelming, and thus prime time for some brain freeze—after all, you are facing living alone in a dorm for the first time in an unfamiliar environment, with new roommates, new schedules, and so on. I tailored this book to the needs of young women during this wonderful but very busy and complex time as a kind of safety handbook, with frank talk, guidelines, resources, advice, and philosophy on a range of issues for the newly independent from campus to Facebook to shopping to self-defense. Please, do me a favor and make the choice to learn how to protect yourself against crime. And remember, caring about your personal safety is not about living paranoid—it is about living smart. It translates into every aspect of your life; it makes you a better student, co-worker, daughter, sister, friend. Trust me, while I would not change a moment of my life and the incidents that have brought me here today, I do not want you ever to experience the debilitating fear and emotional trauma that I have endured from being a victim.

Who Is the Safety Chick?

In November of 1982, I answered a phone call that would change my life forever. On the other end of the line was a former high school acquaintance, who had become fixated on me and decided to make my life a living hell. After the first one, there were many other harassing calls. By a long and perilous process, the situation came down to this man showing up at my door with a semiautomatic weapon and 180 rounds of ammunition. The high (or rather, low) point, ultimately, was his attempting to kidnap me and an eleven-hour police standoff. At the time, there were no laws on the books declaring stalking a felony, and so my official recourse was minimal; every time this person violated a restraining order issued on my behalf, the penalty was just a brief stay in county jail. Over the years, I gained first-hand knowledge of how our legal system works, as well as the trial-by-fire survival skills that one day saved my life.

"What does not destroy me makes me stronger." **—Friedrich Nietzsche**

When the threatening behavior of the stalker—I learned to understand the true meaning of this word—persisted and then escalated, my whole existence came to be consumed by fear and insecurity. In the beginning, I was living in denial, thinking that this guy would go away and everything would return to normal. No such luck. I tried to maintain some semblance of a "normal life" (going to college, participating in activities, building friendships, even getting married), but being pulled by the tension between these two realities was an extremely emotional and exhausting way to live.

One afternoon, I came home from work. Per my routine, I went to the phone, punched a button, and stood listening to the messages on my answering machine. Then I turned around, and found my stalker standing behind me with a knife. This one moment was the culmination of a cat-and-mouse game that had been going on for eight years. My instant reaction was one that surprised both the stalker and me. My first words were, "Sit down, I've been expecting you. We need to talk." My demeanor was calm and in control. I could feel the power shift; I could see a bit of insecurity and nervousness set in, could tell that he was wondering why I was being so unperturbed and apparently hospitable. I realized he was probably expecting me to react with terror, which would make me weak and thereby feed his power and purpose. I truly believe that my cool and confident demeanor got me out of that life-threatening situation physically unharmed. My calmness allowed my stalker to feel comfortable guiding me outside, thus letting his guard down. He did not realize the police had surrounded the house, and in one fell swoop I was able to run away to the waiting arms of a policeman, and he was left in a standoff with the police. They were able to get a handle on the situation and arrest him without anyone getting seriously hurt. This was the start of the Safety Chick mindset: You can make the choice to take control of the fear.

A few months after my confrontation with the stalker, I was contacted by Ed Royce, currently a U.S. congressman and at that time a California state senator who was working on anti-stalking legislation he'd written that would make the crime a felony. He asked if I would testify in front of the state senate. As I sat in front of the committee, recounting each event, I began to feel a power inside me that I had not felt in a long time. It was at that moment that I realized I no longer had to live like a victim. The way to get my power back was to become proactive. This is the second phase of the Safety Chick mindset: Taking control of your own actions gives you inner strength and a sense of empowerment.

In the wake of these experiences, I started speaking at law-enforcement training workshops all over the country. This work introduced me to all kinds of incredible personal-safety and threat-assessment experts and exposed me to their valuable information. I realized that the developments in understanding and strategy needed to get out to the people who could really use it the most: women. Most of the existing personal-safety information circulating seemed to me to be set in a tone and terms to make women feel frightened and overwhelmed, not confident and capable. This is what led to the third phase of the Safety Chick mindset: Being aware of your personal safety should be as routine as brushing your teeth. Implementing personal-safety behaviors should not be an ominous, paranoid, and/or hysterical process, but rather one with a positive, confident attitude combined with lots of common sense.

Finally, what rounds out the mindset of a Safety Chick can be described as the combination of a sense of humor and a sassy edge—something that all college students need to get through your hectic (or even your most mundane) days. Lots of times turning a negative into a positive starts with finding a little bit of humor in the situation; sometimes you need to call on your sense of humor afterward, to help you keep perspective. Either way, humor has great power to get you to the desired end: an empowered attitude!

Use this book as you would a guidebook or reference book. You don't need to read it cover to cover and implement every safety tip all at once. Refer to it as needed: when you first go off to school; when you're preparing to travel or just going to a party in a new scene; when you have questions about using social media on the Internet; when you find yourself in an uncomfortable or potentially unsafe relationship; when you have suspicions about someone in your life. What I want you to take away from it is the overall lifestyle of a Safety Chick: a woman who is confident, empowered, and aware of her surroundings. Throughout the book, you'll find lessons about the choices you must make to stay safe and secure. There will be no pop quiz at the end of each chapter (we get enough of those kinds of tests, big or small, every day of our lives). In the end, you will gain something much more important than any grade or class credit: you will be awarded a strong, positive, and SAFE life.

This book is geared toward young women heading off to or already attending college, and many of the specifics here are pointed to that exciting and challenging time of life. But I also realized as I was writing that, at the end of the day, we are all the same, no matter our age. We are women, navigating through life just at different phases. Heck, it wasn't THAT long ago I was a cheerleader at UCLA, driving around Los Angeles in my convertible Volkswagen bug . . . although the slang might be different, and the clothing styles have changed, and the technology is a bit more advanced, the dangers are still the same. Assault, robbery, stalking, rape. The hard reality is, no matter how old or how young, no matter what shape or size, no matter what skin color or race, we are women, and WOMEN ARE THE NUMBER ONE VICTIMS OF CRIME IN THE WORLD. Now let's work together, you and me, to change this statistic.

*Intuition—
the Key to Personal Safety*

When I was in college, I had a chartreuse Volkswagen bug convertible. It was so bright, it glowed. One day I was driving to downtown LA with the top down. My car stereo had been stolen for the fifth time and I hadn't replaced it yet, so the only way I could listen to music was with a Walkman (that was what we had before iPods—they played CDs, or even cassettes, if you can believe it). So there I was, Miss Thang, driving in a questionable part of town with my car top down, headphones on, and UCLA cheerleading pom-poms in my back seat, completely oblivious to what was going on around me. Thankfully, a policeman had the good sense to pull me over and give me a ticket. (It is against the law to drive with headphones on.) He was not amused by my girlish charms, and rightfully so. After giving me a much-needed scolding, he sent me on my way. As he drove away, I could almost read his mind—"When are these girls going to learn?" Little did I know, I was breaking the most important rule of safety: I was unaware of my surroundings and totally disconnected from my intuition.

Trust Yourself

You hear it time and time again: listen to your gut instinct, your intuition (if only we'd done that with some of our ex-boyfriends, lol). The fact is, it works. If you just take the time to get in tune with your surroundings, you will almost always be able to avoid a negative situation before it happens. Many college students make the mistake of thinking that their campus is just like home—safe and cozy. Because classrooms, dorm rooms, and lounges feel like protected environments, students let their guard down and a lot of times ignore or "turn off" their intuition for fear of being perceived (even if only by themselves) as paranoid or geeky. While these work and living spaces are indeed protected by the institution with the intention of making them happy and healthy refuges, it is a big mistake to forget that they are essentially still public places, and vulnerable to random forces. You *must* use your intuition; it is an essential part of your life. It's like that famous perfect little black dress; without it, your wardrobe is not complete. You cannot even begin to tap into your intuition, however, if you are not aware of your surroundings. Please remember this as you sprint out your door in the morning, late for class, or are coming home from the library late at night and tired from a long session of studying. If you're busy and preoccupied or let fatigue lead to autopilot, how are you going to be able to hear your inner voice? How will you be able to tap into the intuitive body signals that keep you safe from crime?

Again and again, crime victims report that the criminal "caught them by surprise" or "they didn't know what hit them." I cannot impress upon you enough: Taking the time to be aware of your surroundings can save your life. But at the same time, I can't tell you enough: It is not about feeling paranoid, it is about being street smart. Intuition just means acknowledging what you already know inside, recognizing that the "butterflies" feeling in your stomach or the prickly sensation down the back of your neck means your inner bank of signal switches is trying to tell you something. It could be the little voice that says, "Something isn't right," or "This guy is really a creep." Learning to sense your body's intuitive signals is the first step to personal safety.

Tips for Tuning Your Intuition Antennae

The following section offers a few tips to further define intuition and help you learn to exercise all of yours. Think about each of the scenarios described and apply them to your daily life—what would you do? Think them through, play them out in your head, and focus on the feelings that come up to practice getting in tune with your intuition. In addition to the role it plays in safety skills, honing your intuition is good for many, many ordinary moments, too, like choosing a class or whether to go out or stay in. It might even weed out the Mr. Wrongs and improve your love life!

"The only real valuable thing is intuition." —**Albert Einstein**

TIP #1 "SHIVER ME TIMBERS"—Pay Attention When Your Body Gives You Signals

Close your eyes . . . take a deep breath . . . and relax. Don't worry, I'm not going New Age on you—I just want you to *literally* listen to your heart beating and your lungs breathing. Your body does these miraculous things without you even noticing. That's the goal of intuition: to hear your body's signals without even realizing it. You would be amazed at how many things you already do intuitively.

That Knowing Feeling

For example, you're on the beach . . . you're walking down to the water . . . you're in your cute little bikini. What is the first thing you do? You automatically throw back your shoulders and suck in your stomach. That's your intuition, or "gut" instinct (no pun intended), telling you that some hunk on a towel next to you might be checking you out. Now, on a serious note, how about when you're walking down the street and the little hairs on the back of your neck stand up. That's intuition, your body's way of saying, "Something isn't right." Again: Don't ignore that feeling. Take the time to glance behind you or around you. Do you see someone or something that is out of place or a cause for concern? If you do, summon your no-nonsense inner voice that says, "Okay, calm down and don't panic." If you are too busy being scared, you don't have time to think clearly. Is there a store close by that you can go into? Is there a group of people you can stand by? The key is to quickly assess the situation and remove yourself from harm's way.

Chilly Willy

Like that prickling at the back of your neck, if a chill down your spine is not because someone has just dropped an ice cube down your back, it's your intuition at work. For example, this sensation might come over those of you who like to jog on public streets and walkways or on more secluded trails like in parks or nature preserves. If you feel the chill, don't ignore it—it could be someone sneaking up behind you. Don't be embarrassed to turn around or chide yourself for being paranoid. Simply confront the situation; literally turn and take a look. It might be nothing more than the neighbor out walking his dog. But it also could be someone intending to do you harm. If you exercise outdoors, always do so with a friend. If you must exercise alone, be sure to read the self-defense chapter (Bring It On!, page 170) first. Use that chill and your Safety Chick will to thwart a surprise attack or avert a bad choice at one of those proverbial turns in the road or dark alleys. Don't wait for the bad guy to get to you. I repeat: Remove yourself from harm's way.

Butterflies Are Free

Butterflies in your stomach can signal a number of things, but they are an intuitive signal, nonetheless. When you are about to make a presentation in front of your professor or take a test in a classroom, that flapping feeling is your body registering all the tensions and energies in the room as well as your nervousness or excitement, and expressing its response in a physical sensation. In another situation, the reason for the butterflies might be more serious. Instead of flutters, you may feel more of a tightening in your stomach. For example, have you ever entered a party or nightclub and felt that the energy of the crowd seemed to be tense or hostile? That is your intuition telling you that something is about to happen. It could just be the presence of one jerk in the mood to spread some jerkiness around. Sometimes it may mean a fight is brewing, sometimes something worse. Listen to the signal and get out before anything happens.

These are just a few of the common body signals, and you probably recognize them all, either firsthand or through stories. Think about some of your own personal signals in similar situations, and take the time to listen to your body. Look for patterns or times when you thought later, "I *knew* it!" Test yourself the next time you're driving to the market or out walking. The more you learn to identify situations in your daily routine that require you to use your intuition, the quicker you will come to recognize these moments and connect to your intuition effortlessly.

TIP #2 ALL SYSTEMS GO—Use Your Intuition GPS When Driving around Town

Have you ever been driving in your car and been so preoccupied thinking about what you were going to wear to the party that night or all the homework you needed to finish before you went, that when you pulled into the parking spot, you couldn't even remember driving there? That's what I mean by not being aware of your surroundings. Save the daydreaming for when you're hanging on the couch watching *Jersey Shore*. When you are out on the street, you need to have your intuition GPS fully online, your antennae up and working. In driver training class, they tell you not to have your radio volume up so loud that you can't hear the siren of an emergency vehicle. The same is true for letting the volume of the preoccupations in your head drown out your powers of intuition. If you can't hear him coming up beside you—"him" meaning anyone from a gawker looking to make an inappropriate remark to a potential carjacker—when you do finally notice him, it may be too late to avoid unpleasantness or real trouble.

The Window Washer

Has a stranger ever attempted to wash your windshield when you were stopped at a light? If the answer is yes, what was your first reaction? Did you flinch as the person approached your car? If so, that was your intuition telling you that possible danger was approaching. Don't ignore that signal! The same holds true for any stranger who approaches you while you are in the confinement of your car to ask for money or other assistance. While I am, of course, a believer in charities, I don't believe that donating at the street corner is safe. Keep your windows rolled up, lock the doors, and don't make eye contact. Save the contribution for a charity of your choice, such as local shelters or other nonprofits.

You Are Not AAA

If you see a motorist who is broken down or otherwise stranded, your best course is to use your cell phone, report the location to the police, and let them handle it. Your first impulse might be to pull over and help, but your intuition, or in this case, your common sense (the two are closely related) should tell you that the days of helping strangers by the side of the road are over. If you truly feel that the person needs help and you don't have a cell phone, make a note of the car make, license plate number, and location and call the police and report the problem as soon as you get to your destination or find a telephone. This policy doesn't mean that you can't be helpful and compassionate; it just means that you have to act on those impulses in different ways.

Get Off My Tail

Have you ever been driving and noticed that the same car has been behind you for several blocks? What did that *feel* like? Or, what was it that made you notice? Was something inside your brain triggered to make you look in your rearview mirror? Once again, that's your intuition, like an inner lightbulb that goes on alert: "Hey, wait a minute, is someone following me?" Don't ignore the signal. If you think a car is following you, it may be because your intuition picked up on something in its movements that sets it apart from coincidence of traffic patterns. Make a turn and then another, and maybe a third. If the car is still behind you, call 911 on your cell phone and drive straight to the nearest police station. If you do not know where the station is, drive to a really busy area and park safely where there is a flow of people traffic while you wait for the police to arrive. If it's nighttime, make sure it's a brightly lit parking area, such as at a gas station or an open store. Do not lead a criminal to your house or dorm, where he can follow you up your driveway or see where you live.

TIP #3 THE MEMORY GAME—Learning to See Clues

I always use the phrase, "Be aware of your surroundings." I like to use the following simple memory game to turn that concept into a real and concrete learning process. Play it with your roommates. It's a simple exercise: For round one, have your roommate change the location of a few key items in various rooms of your dorm or apartment (choose things that have a usual place), then enter each room and see if you can identify the switches. Knowing what goes where will help you notice immediately if something is amiss at other times; an altered arrangement is a possible sign that an intruder has been there.

For round two, agree with your roommate on some ideas for positioning a few common household objects in places that will betray disturbance. For example, put a flowerpot in front of a window or on a windowsill, and lean a box or package against the outside of the door. Have your roommate move these objects (or not) in an unpredictable way when you're out over the course of a day or two, and try to remember to consciously observe any changes (or lack of them) every time you return to your home.

These simple exercises can do much to sharpen your memory intuition and develop skills for identifying when something is "off." You may want to incorporate parts of the exercises as habit; in the case of a real intruder, you would easily be able to tell if someone had disturbed the flowerpot or knocked over the package, a sign that someone entered, or tried to enter, your room.

If you ever feel that someone other than your roommate has been in your room or apartment, do not go inside. Go to a neighbor's house or stay in your car and dial 911. The police are more than happy to check things out for you, even if you have the smallest suspicion. They would rather have one crime (burglary) to investigate, than two (assault or worse).

TIP #4 USE YOUR RADAR DETECTOR

When you meet someone in a public setting, like the library or gym, for example, have you ever thought, "This person is a little strange" (and not just because he's got teeth like Austin Powers)? That is a great thing you could call intuition radar. An "object" has entered your field, and while it might seem normal enough, your inner voice is saying, "Steer clear." As women, we have in many ways been conditioned to be polite to everyone who crosses our path in a social setting, including some obnoxious men who won't take no for an answer. We are more concerned with being called a bitch than protecting ourselves. Don't worry about being rude or hurting someone's feelings. Many assault victims wish that they had not been so nice to the stranger at the Internet cafe, the food court, the bookstore.

The Eyes Have It

There are many ways to sense if someone is a possible danger to you. A good indication can be found by looking into his eyes. You know the saying: The eyes are the window to the soul. Well, if a person's eyes appear glassy or glazed over, chances are this is not someone you want to be around. Another signal is if the stranger stares at you inappropriately, especially a wide-eyed, intense, or fixed stare. There is an acceptable amount of time that a stranger should look at you. You decide that amount of time with your intuition radar. Once you start to feel uneasy or self-conscious, the stranger should look away. Continued staring should be a red flag.

Space Invaders

When a total stranger asks you for private information, do you feel uncomfortable giving it? Perhaps a department store clerk has asked you for your Social Security number, and you really didn't want to disclose it. That's intuition again, working together with your common sense to say "Now, why would she need to know that?" Many victims of credit card fraud are shocked to find that the criminal was the person at the local store. There is absolute truth to the concept of needing your space, quite literally. Be aware of people standing around you when you are giving out personal information. Likewise, step away when an okay-seeming person seems to be trying very hard to make you trust her; it could well be an identity-theft artist trying to learn your address, telephone number, and Social Security number.

When someone is standing too close behind you, ask yourself a couple of questions. Are you two the only ones at the counter? If so, why is the person standing so close? Is the person paying inappropriate attention to your transaction or does it feel like she is trying to make physical contact? This is not to imply that every nosy person is a criminal (if that were true, all of our boyfriends' moms would be in jail). It's just that you need to be aware of the people around you. If something doesn't feel right, do something about it. Get outta there!

These are just a few examples of how your intuition works. It is up to you to identify your own inner body signals. Practice the exercises and exercise the practices discussed above and see what works for you. When you take the time to practice, noticing the connections and understanding them becomes second nature. Once you start taking responsibility for your own personal safety, you take away the fear of becoming a victim and turn intuition into empowerment. I will go into further detail about what to do after your intuition has signaled your body to act later in the book. Remember: Without using your intuition, all the tips in the world won't help you stay safe from crime.

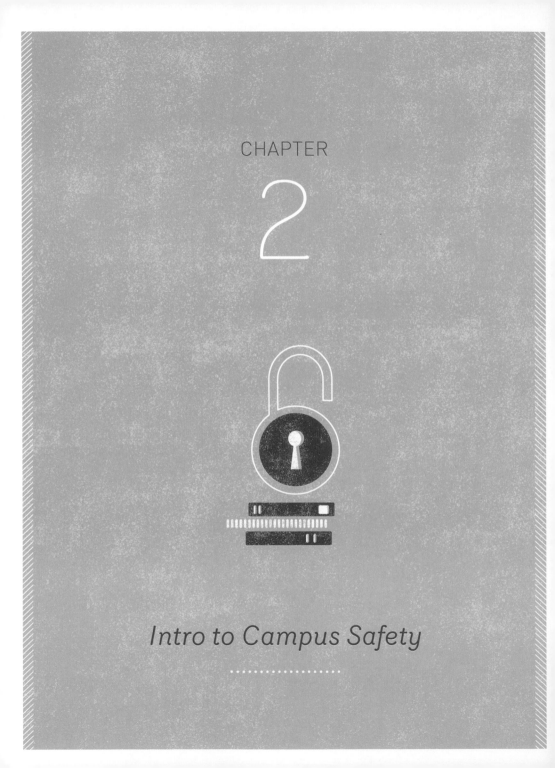

CHAPTER

2

Intro to Campus Safety

Woo-hoo! You finally made it! All the hours of studying in high school, all the sacrifices you have made, all the following of your parents' rules has been worth it: you are now a college student! Nothing compares to that newfound freedom of living on your own— no rules, new friends, and LOTS of parties. Think of it . . . hundreds or even thousands of students just like you, leaving home for the first time, all coming together on one campus. The energy is *amazing*. But it can also be extremely tumultuous. That's why Congress designated September as National Campus Safety Awareness Month. Nicknamed "the Red Zone" for its high incidence of sexual assaults and other crimes, the beginning of the school year is typically the most exciting but can also be the most hazardous.

With parties aplenty, it's a great time to meet new people, make new friends, and experience all the wonderful communities within the college campus. Unfortunately, it's also the time violent crimes are most likely to occur—when students let their guard down, are among strangers, or are drinking. In fact, 95 percent of violent campus crimes are alcohol or drug related.

That's why in this chapter I am going to outline THE most important things to know about campus safety. Spend some time reading through these stories, tips, and statistics and you'll be safer as you embark on this exciting new adventure of being a college student.

Safe Campuses Now

Dana Getzinger Foley is the survivor of a brutal attack near campus during her college days, and because of this has made it her mission to keep students safe from crime, through university and college programs, education, and proactive legislation. She is also the founder (along with her parents Jim and Lisa Getzinger) of Safe Campuses Now, a safety organization they ran for twenty years in Athens, GA.

On a terrible night in 1983, Dana returned home from her sorority's winter formal with her roommates. The evening had been a blast for her. She went to bed, and when she woke up—her life was changed forever. Here is her story.

The Past

"I was asleep on my bed when an intruder broke in through a sliding glass door. I woke up with a pillow over my face. I fought the pillow off and felt a sharp punch in my stomach. It was a knife, which punctured my aorta.

"I remember lying on the floor while one of my roommates held my hand, begging me not to die. I recall a doctor raising my eyelids and hearing a reassuring voice say, 'She's still with us.' It grew harder to stay in tune with the sounds around me. I was afraid to fall asleep. The next thing I remember was my parents' voices and the comfort I felt when they squeezed my hand. I had just undergone extensive surgery to save my life.

"Although I fully recovered, coping with the fears and memories of my attack caused me enormous anguish when I returned to the University of Georgia. Why was I the victim of such an isolated incident? However, my anguish turned to anger when I learned I was one of five students attacked during a two-month period—all within a mile of one another. The other girls had been raped, sodomized, and one girl was stabbed in the back. Weren't students made aware of crimes occurring around them? Why did the statistics I was shown the following year not include any of our attacks? Why aren't crimes against students publicized?

"While my attack may sound violent and brutal, it's an unfortunate reality of the society we live in. Many people have had these experiences, and the reason I am writing about it now is because I want college students to realize how vulnerable they really are."

A New Beginning

"These realities in our society do not make them acceptable. The false sense of security students live under is perpetuated due to the fact that crimes against students are severely underreported.

"A year after my attack, I testified before Congress in support of the Student Right to Know and Campus Security Act, affectionately known as 'The Clery Bill' (see 'It Takes a Village (or Some Really Brave, Strong People) to Make Change,' opposite). This legislation makes it mandatory for colleges and universities to report their crime statistics. Jeanne Clery was murdered in her dorm room at Lehigh University. She was strangled and tortured to death.

"While in Washington, I met the Clerys along with many other parents who all wore buttons with pictures of their children who had been murdered at college. All I could picture was my parents wearing buttons with my picture on them. I suddenly realized how fortunate I was and how serious the problem of crime at college had become. This trip to Washington fueled my motivation to start Safe Campuses Now.

"SCN became a national non-profit organization dedicated to making students more aware and prepared to avoid and deter crime. Through our appearances on various shows and news programs, Safe Campuses Now became the expert on crime against students in the off-campus student community."[1] Safe Campuses Now closed shop in 2009, but its leaders continue to spread Dana's message of personal safety. Katherine "Keith" Sims is taking the organization to a new level and will make all of the content available to students nationwide (see Resources).

Dana's experience was an unusual one, and tragic in its extreme horrors. But her story is not included here to scare you. I include it to remind you that crime can happen everywhere—even on "safe" college campuses. Through Dana's hard work and that of others like her, there are now wonderful campus security programs and organizations that work to keep students safe.

It Takes a Village (or Some Really Brave, Strong People) to Make Change

Before 1990, colleges and universities were not required to report campus crime or security policies. Because of this, a lot of campus crime went "unnotified" and therefore unnoticed by the public . . . until one strong and brave family stepped forward and took matters into their own hands.

In 1986, Jeanne Clery, a college freshman, was murdered in her dorm room at Lehigh University in Bethlehem, Pennsylvania. Jeanne's attacker was a fellow student whom she did not know. The night Jeanne died, the doors to her dorm had been propped open by her fellow dorm mates—a violation of basic safety rules with unintended but terrible results. What is even more troubling about Jeanne's terrible fate is that the university administration was already aware of the threat from the person who would become her murderer; records predating the killing state that the boy had a "proclivity for antisocial behaviors

[1] Dana Getzinger Foley's story copyright © 1990, Safe Campuses Now. Reprinted with permission.

and substance abuse problems." And yet, there were no policies or procedures in place to report the disturbed student's behavior or to make other students aware of possible safety and security issues.

The Clerys took this devastating tragedy and turned it into a mission for change, becoming active in efforts to make all college campuses safer. They created a nonprofit organization called Security On Campus and, along with Dana Getzinger Foley's testimony before Congress, championed the United States' first federal law requiring that colleges and universities keep and disclose information about campus crime and security policies. Under the Jeanne Clery Disclosure of Campus Security Policy and Campus Crime Statistics Act, schools must publish and distribute an annual report that contains three years' worth of campus crime statistics and certain security policy statements, including sexual assault and basic victims' rights policies, the law enforcement authority of campus police, and where students should go to report crime on campus. (For more detailed information on what the reports cover, visit www.securityoncampus.org.)

Federally funded colleges and universities are also required to provide "timely warnings"—a somewhat subjective directive triggered if the administration feels any crime poses an "ongoing threat to students and employees." However, these institutions are also required to keep a separate and more extensive public crime log that keeps track of all incidents reported to the campus police or security department. This log covers all crimes, not just those required in the annual report, such as theft—information that can provide a helpful heads-up or a life-saving alert to students living on or around the campus.

The log must be publicly available during normal business hours, which means that in addition to students and employees, the general public, including parents or members of the local media, have access to it.

There are many excellent Web sites where you can check out crime statistics for your college or campuses you are interested in (see Resources, page 192). Dedicate some time to taking a look, and get familiar with what types of crimes exist or may be prevalent on your campus—it might surprise you. It is not always the large schools that have the most crime; it is not always the smaller campuses that are the safest. Knowledge is power and is the key ingredient to staying safe.

"Courage is not the absence of fear, but rather the judgment that something else is more important than fear." **—Ambrose Redmoon**

What Makes a Campus Safe?

Look, it's hard enough to decide which college is right for you. There are so many factors to consider: Do you want to stay close to home (or as far away as possible); what school has the best program for your major; which school has the cutest guys, and so on and so on. Trying to figure out the safety issues can seem overwhelming. Well, thanks to an extremely talented reporter by the name of Lisa Collier Cool, a lot of your questions have already been answered. Lisa and a team of investigative reporters and security experts compiled for an article in *Reader's Digest* magazine a list of security measures that all college campuses should have in place to create a safe and secure environment for students and faculty. *Reader's Digest* then asked 291 of the top colleges to participate in a survey to assess the safety of their campus. Of those, 135 agreed to supply data (it tells you something about the ones who didn't in the declining itself) for nineteen safety measures, the results of which were then tabulated to construct a tool called the Safety Preparedness Index.

The variables were:

- Number of Students Overall
- Percentage of Students in Dorms with Security Cameras
- Percentage of Students in Dorms with an Attendant (or RA)
- Percentage of Students in Dorms with Full-Time Security
- Percentage of Students in Dorms that Have Rooms with Self-Locking Doors
- Percentage of Students in Dorms with Smoke Detectors on Each Floor
- Percentage of Students in Dorms with Sprinkler Systems
- Has Parking Lots on Campus Monitored by Security Cameras
- Percentage of Campus Protected by Blue-Light Phone (a phone booth with a blue light on top that dials the campus police department directly)
- Must Show ID to Enter Library
- Has a Freshman Orientation Program
- Provides a Binge-Drinking Presentation at Freshman Orientation
- Provides a Drug-Use Presentation at Freshman Orientation
- Includes a Discussion of Rape at Freshman Orientation
- Has an Emergency Response Plan
- Has a Mass Emergency Notification System
- Has an Emergency Lock-Down Plan

- Number of Full-Time University Police
- Has Police with Firearms
- Percentage of Students in Dorms with Peepholes or Chain Locks

When all the data had been collected and analyzed, the participating schools were given a grade of A, B, or C. The results are available online at www.rd.com.

This safety-measure checklist is a great tool for you to use in assessing how safety conscious your school or potential school is. The schools that scored an A grade set an example for excellence in the safety arena and are commended for being ahead of the curve in crime prevention; the schools that scored B's or C's are nonetheless likewise commended for participating in the survey and working to foster awareness and create better safety measures on their campuses.

The Game Plan for the New College Student

Becoming familiar with crime statistics and assessing the Safety Preparedness Index is a great start to making your college experience a fun and safe one. But once you have decided which school is best for you, there is still a set of fundamentals you must follow both on and around your campus to make sure you stay safe. Remember: You are responsible for your own actions. Your choices and behaviors are your own. All the safety measures and stats in the world won't help you if you're not making smart personal-safety choices. Read below for some basic guidelines, tips, tricks, ideas, and attitudes to adopt for your entry into your new life. Once you have completed the action items, such as doing your drive-by and getting all the crucial numbers into your cell phone, you can refer back to this game plan from time to time to assess your personal safety on campus as you go through your daily, sometimes crazy, college life.

Be Camera Shy

Do not let your photo appear with your dorm name, address, phone number, or any other identifying info in campus directories that are available to the public. It is best to stay incognito, especially as a new student—you don't want to be a target for businesses or organizations wanting to sell something or "take advantage" of the newbie. Only you should decide who knows where you live.

Get Oriented

Participate in all freshmen orientations the school has to offer. It's a great way to learn the ins and outs of the campus, from how the systems work to the quickest routes to class. And you'll meet a ton of new people in the process!

Do a Drive-By

Whether you'll be traveling mainly by foot, bicycle, car, or public transit, take some time to get to know your way around. Learn how to get from dorm room to classroom and other parts of campus. Survey it block by block, and familiarize yourself with the immediate surrounding neighborhood, too. Make a mental note of where the blue-light phones—emergency phones that dial directly to security— are located.

It's Good to Share

Let your parents and/or close friends know what your daily schedule is. Give them a copy of your class schedule and activities along with a list of important phone numbers like those of your RA, roommate, and counselor, and any other important contact numbers in case of an emergency.

Get Their Digits

Be sure to program the number of your campus police as well as the local police station into your cell phone. Dialing 911 on your cell phone can sometimes direct you to a regional call station miles away. You will have to explain to them exactly where you are, and then dispatch will contact the police agency that is closest to you. Having your local numbers programmed into your phone not only gets you to the agency you need, but also saves time when every second counts. However, 911 is always the best number to call when you are off campus or not in your local city.

Run with a Pack

Safety in numbers: Don't travel alone, especially at night and in the more desolate parts of campus. Avoid isolated shortcuts no matter how tired you are after a long day of studying. And use the campus shuttle service if provided.

Cruise the Streets

Get a feel for what's happening downtown. Lots of universities have wonderful college towns with great restaurants, coffee houses, etc. But, it is still a town or city . . . be aware of the areas or places that seem to attract the crazy or reckless crowds. Steer clear of those areas on a weekend night when things can get out of control quickly. You don't want to be pulled into something just by being in the wrong place at the wrong time.

Eastside Walk It Out, Westside Walk It Out

No matter where you are, on or off campus, you must always be aware of your surroundings. The more familiar you are with the area, the less you become a target for criminals. Remember: Criminals look for the easiest target—that is generally someone who is preoccupied, unsure, and unaware of who or what is around them. Always walk with confidence, like you know where you are going; that's what I call the Safety Chick Swagger.

New Kids on the Block

Remember: If you are in a new town, it may show. The town is filled with people who are strangers to you, but at the same time, you are very familiar to them. When you and your new roomie go to Walmart or Target for your brand-new matching bedding and stuff, be aware of the people around you; criminals in college towns are on the lookout for the newbies to victimize. Be sure no one is following you when you shop or when you head back to your dorm or apartment.

Dark Corners of Campus

Even though this chapter is about campus safety, I want to emphasize that crime against college students is not just perpetrated by other students and does not happen just on campus. You must remember that no school is a closed school. There are thousands of nonstudents who cruise on and off campus every day and night.

It is very important to note that a lot of colleges and universities do not include parking garages in their reporting of campus crime statistics, whether on campus property or in town near campus lines; therefore, there is no way to be sure of the crimes that occur in those places. A dark parking lot can be an unsafe environment, so I want to share these vital tips for when you are parking on campus and around town:

- Park in the lots on campus, as opposed to spaces on side streets or lots downtown. Campus police patrol these areas, making them safer.

- Try to park in a highly trafficked area, not in a dark corner in the back of the garage.
- As you pull into the garage, scan the area for anything or anyone suspicious.
- Think ahead—park in a well-lit area if you plan on coming back to your car after dark.
- Lock your car. Do not use a remote to unlock (or start the motor, if you happen to have a remote engine starter) until you are at your car door— you don't want your attacker or car thief to get to your unlocked door first.
- If you have to use an isolated parking lot, always arrive when you know other students will be there, both at the beginning and the end of your evening. Better yet, always try to use the good old buddy system for your party—the truth of safety in numbers never gets old.
- Have your keys ready before you reach your car.
- Have your cell phone out and ready to use in case of emergency, but wait until you are in a safe location to start chatting with friends.
- Have your backpack or purse on your shoulder(s), keeping your hands and arms free—that way, you are ready to react if someone approaches.
- NEVER leave your keys in the ignition. I have watched people leave their car running and door unlocked while they run into a convenience store or post office, thus presenting the perfect opportunity for car thieves!
- Never leave valuables in plain sight—be sure to lock them in the trunk, hide them under the seat, or stash them in the console or glove compartment.
- Don't leave any paperwork showing personal information, such as your mail, bills, or residential parking permit, visible on the seat or dashboard— you don't want to reveal your name or address to criminals by allowing them to read through your car window.

Taking the time to be alert and aware while getting from point A to point B is the key. Many crimes have happened to people who were distracted and not paying attention to their surroundings. I have watched countless surveillance videos of purse snatchers, abductors, and car thieves brazenly attacking their victims in parking lots and garages. The common thread was that the victims were completely unaware of who was around them and what was happening until it was too late. So the next time you're running to the mall for that great shoe sale, remember to take a moment to park safely and be aware of your surroundings going both to and from (hopefully with a few new pairs of cute stilettos) the store.

What Should You Do? Survival Strategies in the Event of a School Shooting

None of us can forget the horrors of Columbine, Virginia Tech, and other school shooting tragedies. While the odds of a student becoming a victim of a car accident, a burglary, an assault, or even rape are much, much higher, this crime, though so rare as to be still almost unthinkable, is at the forefront of concern and must be prepared for in responsible safety training.

As I have said before, the Safety Chick lifestyle is to think ahead and have a plan. Do not wait until you're in a life-threatening situation to try to figure out what to do. I am a member of the International Association of Chiefs of Police (IACP), an organization that is dedicated to professionalism in law enforcement. Every year police chiefs and law enforcement officials from all over the country converge to network and learn the latest techniques in policing and crime prevention programs. This year I sat in on an excellent presentation on how to prevent mass-casualty shootings. The three presenters were University of Wisconsin police chief Susan Riseling, University of California at Davis police chief Annette Spicuzza, and forensic physiologist Dr. John Nicoletti. I was amazed to hear how law enforcement and school officials all over the country have come together to take action on how to respond to, and possibly prevent, this particular tragedy from happening. In the following section, I have tried to distill the solid and powerfully useful information I learned that day, along with material from the University of Wisconsin, Madison, police department and their commission, who put together the program and created the report. For more information, go to www.uwpd.edu. (BTW, both of the university police chiefs are women—very competent, respected, cool cops who are dedicated to keeping students safe from crime. They are the true meaning of Safety Chicks!)

Prevention and Intervention

After every mass killing in the United States, the subsequent investigations showed that there were warning signs. In the words of Robert Fein of the U.S. Secret Service: "There is always a path to murder." I think what he means by this is that no one just "snaps." A person doesn't wake up one morning and become a shooter. In the case of Columbine, a few students gathered on the second-floor balcony above the library—they had heard through the grapevine that some type of disturbance was planned. At Virginia Tech, many people had reported the soon-to-be shooter's strange behavior both in and outside of the classroom.

The point is, in order to prevent an attack of this terrible and complicated nature, people must learn how to identify signs of a person in crisis and what is the best way to intervene. The list below contains some of the most obvious, and though it is by no means complete, it will arm your awareness. Let me be very clear: This does NOT mean to take matters into your own hands and confront a potentially violent person if you do observe someone displaying one or a number of these symptoms. What it does mean is be observant, and then use the proper channels for reporting suspicious behavior at once.

Possible Signs of a Person in Crisis

- **Chronic depression or mood swings**—We all have our moments of moodiness, but take notice of a person who goes from up to down, happy to sad, angry to nice, erratically and consistently.
- **Perception of injustice**—Someone who has the feeling that someone or everyone has done them wrong, or "the system" is out to get him.
- **Isolating behavior, hostility**—Someone who is a self-described loner, or worse, an angry loner who keeps to him- or herself.
- **Low self-esteem, excuses, blaming**—Someone who feels inferior to everyone else, makes up excuses for his perceived failures, or complains consistently about other people or things; has, as the expression goes, a chip on his shoulder.
- **Strained relationships**—A person who never seems to get along with anyone and has a tumultuous or nonexistent relationship with family and/or friends.
- **Reduced motivation**—Someone who doesn't seem to have the same drive he had before; a lack of energy or interest in things.
- **Changes in health or hygiene**—A formerly normally healthy and tidy person who suddenly starts to show up unshaven or disheveled, like he just rolled out of bed, paying no attention to his appearance or hygiene.
- **Substance abuse**—A person who demonstrates excessive drinking or drug abuse.
- **Frequent allusions to violence**—Someone who has an unhealthy interest in violence or death, talking about weapons and destructive and/or violent behavior in an eager or obsessive way.

If someone you know exhibits some of these signs and you think he might be in crisis, there are things you can to do to help assess the situation. First and foremost, it is important to remain calm. Do not act nervous or accusatory toward the person. For all you know, he or she could just be having a bad week and not dealing with things well. Second, actively listen. It is important to hear and understand where the person is coming from. Listening carefully will help you know if it's a bad week or if the behavior is more serious. Try to communicate and be understanding; you might learn more about the person and why he feels the way he does. Be respectful and patient as you listen. Often, these people feel that they are not being heard, and frustrations can develop from that. If you feel that the person is in crisis, you must set clear boundaries with him. Never make promises you can't keep, and do not attempt to become his therapist.

If you are concerned, do not ignore the signs. Document your observations and tell a trusted RA, teacher, or other professional in the community. If you begin to feel that a person is truly in crisis and a danger to himself or others, it is of utmost importance that you contact a wide field of people for guidance: teachers, RA, the dean of students, the police department, the Student Counseling Center, and any department associated with the school authorities. Remember: Nobody just snaps. Understanding and recognizing the signs of a person in crisis and getting help can lead to an intervention BEFORE something happens.

As I said before, the odds of being a victim of a shooting at school are extremely low, but it still is important to have a plan and viable strategies to use in your time of need. Research shows that if you have thought in advance about what you would do in the event of a mass-casualty incident, your chance of survival is greatly improved; it could be the difference between life and death.

What to Do in the Event of an Active Shooter

As I learned in the mass-casualty shooting presentation (see page 30), if you are ever faced with this very unlikely—and, of course, shocking—event, if you can remember one word, it should be OUT! Here is what they taught us:

Get Out: Run!!
The best option is ALWAYS to run, GET OUT, get away. Think in advance about how you would get out, including the possibility of jumping from the windows.

Call Out: Call 911
If possible, take care of your safety first. Run first, hide first, barricade or lock the door first, then call 911. If it's safe, stay on the line and give the police the best information you can.

Hide Out: Or Play Dead

If you are not able to get out, find a safe place to hide. If there's no way to get out or hide, playing dead could save your life. If you are hiding when the police come, realize they will not know if you're a victim or a shooter. Follow their instructions.

Keep Out: Keep the Shooter Out

If you can't get out, lock or barricade the door. Make sure the barricade stays in place, holding it from a safe position if necessary—many at Virginia Tech survived by securing doors to keep the shooter out.

Take Out: Fight the Shooter

Fight or flight? Flight, running, getting out is ALWAYS the best option. But if flight is removed as an option, your only choice may be to fight. See the self-defense chapter (page 170) to learn more about how to face this extreme situation.

As a general practice, when you go into a situation where you are sharing a closed-in space with a group, such as classrooms, meeting rooms, libraries, immediately give your surroundings a once-over. Observe where the exits are. Look to see if the doors can be locked. Check to see if/how the windows open. Have a plan of action: Where would you run? What would work as a door barricade and how would you hold the barricade? How far is it to the ground if you had to jump out the window? Would you survive the fall? Share this information with your fellow students; discuss what you would do in an emergency.

Bottom line if you are caught in a shooting: Remember the word OUT

GET OUT • CALL OUT • HIDE OUT

KEEP OUT • TAKE OUT

The threat of school shootings can be avoided if everyone works together to identify people in crisis and notify the proper authorities so that an intervention can take place *before* the escalation to violence. Share the OUT strategy with all of your friends and classmates. Knowledge is power and the more people who know how to react in a crisis, the more the crisis can be avoided. You can learn more at the Center for Personal Protection and Safety (see Resources, page 192).

Safety Chick Checklist:
Key Tips for Campus Safety

☒ RESEARCH CAMPUS CRIME STATISTICS

Inform yourself on how your campus rates and where weak spots may lie.

☒ GET FAMILIAR WITH ALL PARTS OF CAMPUS

Tour the lay of the land with a group so you feel confident and are less likely to get lost.

☒ KEEP PERSONAL INFORMATION PRIVATE

Do not let your photo with dorm name, address, phone number, or any other identifying info be put in public directories.

☒ GET ORIENTED

Participate in all the orientations the school has to offer.

☒ KNOW BEFORE YOU GO

Study the routes between your residence and classes or activities, including the location of blue-light security phones.

☒ SHARING IS GOOD

Make a copy of your class/activities schedule and a list of pertinent phone numbers for your parents and a network of close friends.

☒ PROGRAM NEW DIGITS

Put the numbers of your campus security and local city police departments in your cell phone.

☒ RUN WITH A PACK

Travel in groups as much as possible, avoid low-traffic or isolated paths, and use a shuttle service after dark.

✖ BE YOUR OWN P.I.

Research the campus to make sure that buildings, walkways, quadrangles, and parking lots are secured, lit, and patrolled. Make sure that emergency phones, escorts, and shuttle services are actually available, working, and adequate.

✖ TAKE SAFETY TO THE STREETS

To gauge your new social scene, gather a group and stroll through student hangouts. Are people behaving responsibly? Carefully evaluate off-campus student apartment complexes and fraternity houses, too.

✖ EASTSIDE WALK IT OUT, WESTSIDE WALK IT OUT

No matter where you are, always be aware of your surroundings. Always walk with confidence to avoid looking like an easy target—use the Safety Chick Swagger.

✖ NEW KIDS ON THE BLOCK

Remember that criminals have a sharp eye for newbies setting up their lives on campus. Make sure that no one follows you home from trips to the administration building, housewares store, etc.

CHAPTER

3

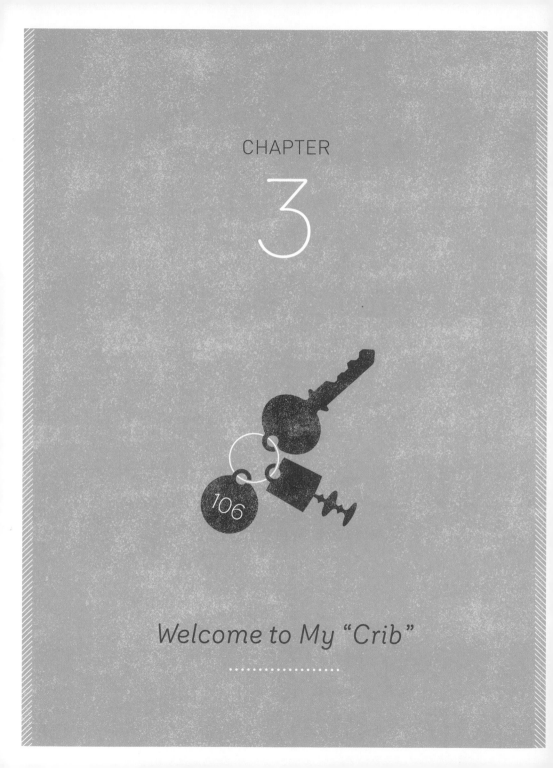

Welcome to My "Crib"

A Southern California college student wanted to stay at school for the summer. Her roommate was leaving to go back home, so in order for her to stay in their apartment, she needed someone to move in for three months to split the rent. She was referred to a friend of a friend, and without much research or background checking, she let this young woman move in. Things seemed okay at first. The new roommate was a beautiful blonde with a killer body and was always dressed in sexy and expensive designer clothing. The student did find it a little odd that the beautiful woman kept really late hours and always had an abundance of cash. . . . That is, until one morning when she caught the new roomie sneaking a middle-aged man out the front door—it was then that she came clean. You see, the beautiful new roommate was not a college student, she was a high-class escort!

Okay, we've all seen those crazy reality TV shows like MTV's *The Real World* and *Big Brother*, where a bunch of strangers move to a new city and live together in some fantastic huge house. While a lot of ridiculous and strange things go on, the REALITY is that that is not reality. Going to college, moving into a new dorm or apartment, and moving in with a complete stranger take more patience, compromise, and compassion than a twelve-week stint on a movie set. This chapter covers Dorm Life 101—we'll discuss dorm-safety guidelines that every college student should follow, vital tips for getting along with your roommates, safety and security rules for living off campus, and ways to keep your possessions from getting ripped off.

Dorm Safety: This Is Not Your Mama's House!

One of the biggest mistakes you can make is thinking that your dorm is an extension of the home you just came from. Just because there is some type of security lock or guard at the front door does not mean that the two-story, two-hundred-room structure is safe from crime. In fact, the large, transient environment of a dormitory is perfect for allowing a person with criminal intent to blend in unnoticed with the comings and goings of what may be hundreds of students living there, not to mention all of their visiting friends. So, study the safety guidelines in the sections that follow, and teach your dorm mates and other friends what you learn. As in other communities, when everyone in a dorm takes on a "neighborhood watch" approach, it goes far toward keeping your dorm safe from crime.

There are three very important rules you must always abide by to create a perimeter of safety around your "crib." Or, in the words of my son Landon: "Put a moat around your castle." These three rules apply even when you are out of college, living on your own, or raising a family. Remember these words: respect, lock, and report.

Respect

When entering your residence hall or building area, you must respect the access-code rules. Think of it this way: Would you let a complete stranger walk into your house with you? Then why let someone without access to your building inside to freely roam around? How awful would you feel if you accidentally let a stalker, thief, or rapist into your dorm and he did harm to a fellow student? Do not worry about being impolite or rude by not letting him in without the proper access; it is the person not respecting the rules who is the rude one.

Lock

Make sure you lock your doors and windows when you leave your room. I know it might be a pain in the you-know-what to lock your door every time you run down the hall to take a shower or see your neighbor. But again, how bad would you feel if while your roommate was at class, you went down the hall to visit your neighbor and came back to find your unlocked door open and your roommate's computer gone! The easiest thing to do is always carry your key with you around the dorm—try one of those bracelet-style stretchy key chains that go around your wrist. Then your keys are always accessible and easy to take with you—even to the shower. Lock your windows as well, especially if you live on the first or second floor. You DO NOT want someone crawling into your room through your window whether you're there or not! Get a window lock at a hardware store that prevents a window from being opened more than a few inches (see Resources, page 192). That way, you can get fresh air without getting unwanted visitors.

Report

Report all suspicious behavior to your residence director or the campus or city police department. Being alert and using common sense is the best way to prevent crime. If something doesn't feel right, if a person seems to be out of place or acting funny, take note. Observe where that stranger is going, what he looks like, what he is wearing. Again, listen to your gut and contact someone of authority. How great would you feel if you took action and actually prevented a crime from happening?

In addition to the three overarching rules above, here is a longer list of very important safety tips specifically for living in a dorm or residence hall.

No Piggybacks

Piggybacking is the perpetrator's oldest form of gaining entry into a secured living space. Oftentimes they will be holding something in their hands (i.e., boxes, flowers, food delivery) and come up right behind you. This leads any decent, honest person to hold the door open for them, at which point they walk right into any part of the secured living space. Thus, they breach the perimeter of safety and gain access to a vast number of innocent targets to prey upon. Once inside, other residents assume that they are there with granted access. It is your duty and obligation to your fellow students to instruct strangers to use the proper access protocol.

You Were Not Raised in a Barn

Just as you would not leave your front door open to the street in the home you came from (unless you lived on a twenty-acre farm in Iowa, and even then, your mama would make you shut it before all the bugs and critters came in), you should not leave your front door open in your dorm room. Even if you are home studying or hanging out, you still need to control who comes into your room and who doesn't. Also, NEVER prop open a door. That goes for any door—to your room, the bathroom, fire doors, and especially the main entrance to the building.

Take a Peep

Hopefully, your door has a peephole. If not, always ask who is at the door before you open it. If you don't know who it is or why they are there, DO NOT OPEN THE DOOR! Use common sense. If you did not order a pizza to be delivered, do not open the door for, "Pizza Man!" If your phone is not broken, do not open the door for someone who says he's the phone repair guy! If you don't or your roommate does not have a friend named Jason, do not open the door for the guy who says, "Hey, it's Jason, open the door!" I bet you are you starting to get the idea. YOU are in control of who comes into your room. YOU don't want to invite danger in. YOU have every right to make the decision to not open the door. A special note: even if the person seems okay, if he is too persistent, that should raise a red flag with you. Call the residential assistant or police for help at once.

Need Help? Yell, Don't Scream

Many security experts warn that in a dorm, screaming can sound like partying. A cry for help may sound like horsing around. Instead, if you need to call for assistance, yell as loudly as you can and use a specific word, like "Help!" "Police!" or "Fire!"

Be Alarming!

There are many wireless and portable systems and gadgets that can secure your room (see my Safety Chick Door Wedge Alarm, for example, in Resources, page 193). There are window and front door contacts/alarm systems that come in easy-to-install do-it-yourself packages. There are even systems that have motion detectors that will send an alert to your cell phone or computer with live audio/video footage of the intrusion. Bottom line: Criminals look for the easy target; a chick with an alarm system in her dorm room is nothing to mess with.

Going Up?

If your dorm has an elevator, use it with awareness. If you are preparing to get in and someone or something in there feels wrong, do not enter (see Chapter 1, "Intuition"). When you do board, stand next to the controls. You want to be in control of the buttons, not the creepy guy who could press the STOP switch. If someone steps on who creeps you out, if you have time, step off right away. If you don't, press a button and get off on the next floor.

Where There's Smoke . . .

Fire safety is a huge problem in dorms around the country. There have been some tragic incidents of serious injury and death from fires in dorms. Make sure your dorm room and hallways have working smoke detectors. Get familiar with your fire escape route. Practice emergency escape routes with your roommate. Don't leave candles or cigarettes burning unattended. Better yet—don't smoke at all!! (Okay, that's the mom in me coming out.) Anyway, take the time to think and care about fire safety. Although firemen may be extremely cute, a better place to appreciate them is hanging on your wall in a monthly calendar, not responding to a fire in your dorm that you might have accidentally set!

Who's on the List

Have a list posted by your front door of emergency numbers. This should include the residential assistants in your building or the resident manager of your dorm, campus police, local police (non-emergency number), your mom and dad's cell and home numbers, your roommate's mom and dad's cell and home numbers, and any close relative or friends that you and your roommate would have on an emergency list. These numbers should be front and center—right alongside the twenty-four-hour pizza delivery service.

Why Can't We Be Friends?
How to Get Along with Roommates

I am sure when you were growing up, you heard stories from your parents, friends, or relatives about their college roommates. Some are best friends for life and some have horror stories to tell. Any way you slice it, roommates have a big impact on your college experience.

At most colleges, freshman roommates are assigned. Once you are an upperclassman, you can request your roommates and get in a pool or drawing for a residence hall or dorm. The way most universities assign roommates is usually based on information the student has provided in a housing/orientation form. According to most campus housing offices, matching up potential roommates is based on a few general things: smoking, alcohol consumption, bed times, study habits, and hobbies. (Like I said before, I wish you wouldn't do it at all, but, smoking is a big issue. Most dorms do not allow smoking inside, but the habit itself can warrant big problems between smokers and nonsmokers.) The second part of the pairing is assessing living habits: cleanliness and messiness. Believe it or not, studies show that even the best of friends have a hard time getting along if one is neat and the other is . . . well, not.

To be sure, check with your housing office to see how they assign roommates, and make sure that all the information you provide is truthful and in-depth and communicates what your likes and dislikes really are. This enables them to pair you with someone with whom you are relatively compatible. That being said, there is no guarantee your new lifelong BFF will walk through that dorm room door and all will be right with the world! The reality of the situation is that to really have a great relationship with your roommate, you must practice the three C's: communication, compassion, and compromise.

Communication

Most colleges give you the name and number of your roommate a few weeks before you start school. Take that opportunity to give her a call. Start by asking her (not grilling her) about herself: what's her home town like, does she have siblings, what does she like to do, and what she wants to study at school. Take an interest in who she is and what she likes, and enjoy getting to know the stranger you are about to hear snore for the next year! Seriously, honest communication about likes and dislikes is important in any healthy relationship. Without honest communication, small issues can get blown out of proportion and then drama will surely ensue.

Compassion

Let's face it: most of your friends up until now have grown up in the same town as you. You all basically have the same background, childhoods, and life experiences. Some might even have known you since kindergarten! When you enter college, you will find that a lot of your dorm mates have had very different childhoods, have grown up in different parts of the country, and have different religious beliefs. But the most important thing to remember is that everyone deserves compassion and respect. Take the opportunity to learn about different cultures and beliefs. One of my first roommates was Jewish. JoAnne and her wonderful family introduced me to bagels, blintzes, matzo balls, and lots of other Jewish foods that I enjoy to this day. I am sure you have heard the old saying, "Treat people the way you want to be treated." Well, it's true, and as long as you operate with that in mind, you and your roommate should be fine.

Compromise

Okay—this is a hard one. But again, if you have any desire to get married down the road, "compromise" needs to become your middle name. If two people are to live together peacefully, there are many things that need to be compromised on. Going to bed at the same time, leaving the light on or off, and having music off or on are all issues that require compromise. For example: if your roommate is a night owl and you're an early-bird-catches-the-worm-type chick (no pun intended), you will need to discuss schedules and come up with a plan. Maybe three nights a week she goes down to the lounge to study while you hit the hay early. On the days you don't have school or an early class, bedtime can be a bit later. Either way, without compromise on BOTH sides, the relationship will never work.

If you find that you and your roommate have aspects of sharing a living space that require a compromise, you must then try to negotiate.

Negotiating a Compromise

Negotiating can be tough, so I've included some professional tips for creating a set of written agreements that can help you through the process. (See Resources, page 197, for a sample roommate agreement.)

According to the experts at Residentassistant.com, putting agreements and understandings in writing helps to clarify issues and provides a point of reference if future conflicts arise. There are many different things you can put down in your agreement. You can create a schedule that carves out when you both will study, what time you agree to go to bed during the week, how late you stay out on weekends. They even suggest that you can create parameters of when each of you can have friends over, or even how loud you can play music. Bottom line is that the more issues and information you can get out on the table to be worked out, the less misunderstanding and conflict will arise.

Understand that sometimes you might not be able to work things out by yourselves. That's why it is important to know that your residential assistant, advisors, or someone in the counseling office is available to help. One last word of advice: do not involve friends or neighbors in your dispute; it just brings more unnecessary drama and conflict into the situation. If you need third party help, seek out a professional.

Be Possessive of Your Possessions: How Not to Get Your Stuff Ripped Off

If you're lucky, for your high school graduation maybe you'll get (or you got) a new laptop, an iPod complete with docking station, some new clothes, or even fabulous bling! You also will probably want to pack it all up and take the new goods with you to college. Well, that will make them perfect pickings for every con artist and thief on and around your college campus. Some universities estimate that more than $100,000 worth of property and equipment is stolen annually from the campus.

If it seems like it would take a den or even two or three dens of thieves to accomplish all that crime, remember that thieves don't necessarily look like thugs—they could be your neighbor down the hall, her friend visiting from home or from another dorm, or a nonstudent well disguised as one. So take these necessary precautions to keep your stuff safe.

Make It Personal

Engrave your valuable items with your driver's license or student ID number so police can track them if they are stolen. Some police stations even have free engraving machines you can borrow.

Get Insured

Get renter's insurance to cover all your valuable possessions. Check with your family's insurance agent. Your family homeowner's policy might already cover the contents in your apartment or dorm.

Safeguard

Get a small safe to keep your valuable jewelry, cash, and other items in.

Take a Picture, It'll Last Longer

Take photos of all your valuables and store them on a photo CD along with a detailed list; leave a copy at home with your parents for safekeeping.

You Are Not A-1 Rents

Do not loan your valuables to your friends or roommates. Your generosity is to be commended, but unfortunately, you can't control who uses and takes care of your stuff once it's in someone else's hands.

You CAN Take It with You

Take all of your valuables home with you for weekend breaks and vacations.

Lock It Up

Get good solid locks for your bike or scooter. The sturdy U-shaped titanium locks (Kryptonite is the ubiquitous brand) work best—be sure to put the lock through the frame and a wheel, if possible (an additional cable helps for this), and lock it to a sturdy bike rack. For computers and other electronics or things of value that you carry with you around campus, there are great portable locks that have alarms on them that attach to a security strap with a pull pin. If the strap is detached, a loud siren will sound, drawing attention to the thief! (See Resources, page 192.)

The key is to carefully keep track of your valuables and not to flash them around your dorm, library, classrooms, or common areas. Word gets around of who has what and thieves love to target those with the good goods.

Outside the Box: Living Off Campus

Making the decision to live off campus in a house or apartment is a big deal. It is mostly upperclassmen who make the move. One or two years in a dorm can get old for some students and the idea of moving off campus for more freedom and independence sounds exciting.

Some of my best memories at UCLA were of living with five roommates in a huge apartment a few blocks away from campus. It was so fun creating our own home, with our own kitchen, living room, dining room, and bedrooms. Trips to Target and Walmart for home décor items were awesome. For the most part, everyone got along and things went smoothly. But every once in a while, a late payment of bills, trash not taken out, dirty dishes in the sink, someone's six-pack of Diet Coke gone missing, could stir up a bit of unrest. What I know now—and wish I had done then—is that it is important to take the time to create that "common ground" I talked about in the section on dorm life (see page 41). It is even more important to get things in writing in a rental partnership; that's because entering into a lease for an apartment or house is a legally binding contract between you and a landlord. Every one of your roommates must be on board with the lease requirements, since whoever's name is on that lease is legally responsible for that contract. So before you throw your stuff in a box and say *"Adios!"* to dorm life, here are a few things to consider, courtesy of CollegeBoard.com:

The Pros of Living Off Campus

- **Saving some dough**—Sometimes living off campus with a bunch of roommates to offset the rent can be cheaper than university housing.
- **No more community bathrooms**—You'll have more privacy and space, and you won't need to wear sandals when you take a shower.
- **Quiet time**—Private apartments are usually quieter and have fewer distractions, and therefore are better for studying.
- **Helps develop credit**—Establishing financial credit through paying your rent and utility bills on time will help you enter the real world more efficiently.
- **No more meatloaf, peas, and carrots**—Buying your own groceries and making your own meals is a big improvement on dorm food.

The Cons of Living Off Campus

- **Spending more dough**—If you are moving out by yourself or just one roommate, the rent can be much higher than living on campus. Utility bills, grocery bills, and household stuff like cleaning supplies, etc., all add up pretty quickly if you aren't splitting with a big group. And don't forget all the furniture and housewares you will need to set up an unfurnished place.

- **Less convenience**—Unless you are a trust-fund baby, you will not have the luxury of a cleaning service—you will need to slap on those rubber gloves and clean your own bathroom. You will also spend more time running to the grocery store and other errands if you live off campus.

- **It's lonely**—Living off campus can get a little lonely. On campus, there is always someone around to study with or grab a bite to eat with. With no one around, you might feel a bit isolated.

- **School's out for the summer**—If you sign a yearlong lease, it ties you to staying at school through the summer. If you want to go home, you have to find someone to sublet for a few months, which can be complicated (if your landlord even allows it).[2]

These lists are just to get you thinking. Sit down and create your own pro and con lists of things that are important to you. Also, do a side-by-side comparison of all the expenses involved with living on campus versus off campus.

If you have decided to take the plunge and live off campus, visit the off-campus housing office at your school. This is where you can find housing, landlord, management company, and roommate listings. Note that most off-campus housing offices do not inspect the housing options they list—that is your responsibility. The office can give you advice on the best time to conduct your search, what to do if you encounter discrimination in your housing search, and how to resolve differences with your landlord or fellow tenants. Remember: NEVER go look at an apartment or house by yourself. Bring along your roommate or a friend—safety in numbers. Also check your campus and local newspaper, Craigslist, and other sites like Apartmentguide.com and Move.com for housing listings.

[2] Pro and con list from *Thinking of Living off Campus?* copyright © 2010 by The College Board. Reprinted with permission. http://www.collegeboard.com/student/csearch/campus-life/9870.html

Safety Chick Checklist:
What Defines a Safe Building?

Much like the safety guidelines for living in the dorms, building access and security are top priorities when looking for an apartment or housing complex. Here is a checklist to help you make a safe pick when house hunting.

✖ I AM THE GATE KEEPER
Security access is required for entry: key card, codes, front desk security, etc.

✖ LOCK, STOCK, AND DEADBOLT
Exterior doors are equipped with sturdy deadbolts and locks.

✖ A WELL-LIGHTED PLACE
Exterior lighting is bright and effective all the way around the building twenty-four hours a day.

✖ PARK HERE
Parking lots and structures are extremely well lit and have security cameras or guards monitoring them.

✖ NO COVER OF DARKNESS
Laundry rooms and common areas like lobbies, pools, and courtyards are well lit, require secure access, and are fitted with security cameras.

✖ NO ENTRY, YES EXIT
All side doors and emergency exits are secured from the inside and locked from the outside, but easy to exit from in case of fire or other emergency.

✖ JUST THE RIGHT HEIGHT
Choose a unit located between the second floor and sixth floor, high enough so intruders can't readily climb through windows but low enough so a fire ladder can reach them in case of emergency (see page 108).

✖ SMOKE BANDITS
Smoke detectors are installed and working properly throughout the building and your unit.

✖ PRIORITY POST
Mailboxes are in a secured, well-traveled area and have solid locks on each box.

Be Ahead of the Game

Remember, there is always a lot of competition for finding that choice apartment and location, especially before the beginning of school or the start of a semester. The more prepared and ready to go you are, the better chance of landing the apartment you want.

Start the hunt as early as possible

Begin looking at least a month before the start of the semester. While you're looking, stay with friends or family or in a hotel—in other words, you will need time to find the place that is right for you.

Have your cash ready

You will need a check or cash (preferably a check to have documentation or proof of the deposit). Be sure to get a receipt from the landlord or property manager.

Provide the necessary documentation

Usually in order to qualify to rent an apartment, you will need to provide several pieces of information. If you don't have the required information, you will need either your parents or a guardian with you to co-sign. They will have to provide a copy of their previous year's tax return, recent pay stubs, personal and business references, contact information from previous landlords if applicable, and photo identification.

Signing a Lease = Serious Commitment

Before you sign ANYTHING, you must read it extremely carefully and be absolutely ready to commit (that goes for a marriage proposal as well, lol). A lease is a binding, legal contract between you and your landlord. It outlines the rights and responsibilities of both parties. It is imperative that both you and your parents, any roommates who are going to co-sign with you, and their parents read the contract thoroughly and agree to everything that is on there BEFORE you sign. Staff at your college's off-campus housing office might also be able to look over the contract or the lease and give you advice if you have any questions.

Put on Your Power Hat and Negotiate!

Don't be afraid to negotiate any part of the lease with your landlord. Remember, your landlord is only obligated to provide services explicitly stated in your lease and under the housing laws. So, if you have negotiated any extra items—like new carpet to be put in by landlord before move-in date, or landlord to pay utilities—be sure to get it in writing IN THE LEASE CONTRACT.

Renter Beware

There are abundant how-to-do-its available for prospective renters. From my own experience, however, dating back to my college days in Southern California, I have assembled a few cardinal rules:

- Before you sign a lease, make sure you understand the terms for renewal or termination. Can you sublet? How do you reclaim your security deposit? How long after you move out do you get your money back? Will your landlord keep any of your deposit for cleaning/painting/etc.? Personal testimony: hungry landlords have withheld hundreds of dollars from my deposits on a variety of specious excuses. Specifics must be clearly outlined in the contract. After lease termination, it's too late.

- Be careful of "riders." Do you understand what a "rider" is? Well, it is an amendment to a contract or policy. Don't let any riders in the lease slip by. It could be something written in by the landlord, such as: "Tenant is responsible for all utilities—even the water for the outside of the property" (which should NOT be a tenant's responsibility if it is a duplex or an apartment complex). Any riders are binding, just like the language in the lease itself.

- Group rentals, common among students, are advisable only when all participants are named in the lease. Ideally, every tenant should sign a separate lease. Make sure you're not holding the bag if a roommate skips out without adequate payment.

- Ask about repairs. It is crucial that you clearly understand the types of modifications that fall within the responsibility of both you and the landlord. Make sure you fully understand what you are allowed to change—even if you think you are making the landlord's unit look better, it might end up costing you more in the end.

For any other questions or issues that may arise, the best place to find out your rights as a renter is the U.S. Department of Housing and Urban Development, www.hud.gov.

Snug as a Bug: How to Secure Your Home Inside and Out

Once you have found your "killer crib," along with the new couches, tables, lamps, and all that fun stuff you require, there are a few security accessories that you will need, as well as a checking-it-twice checklist and a few basic renter's rules to engage. Making your home safe and secure allows you to feel "snug as a bug in a rug" and enjoy those long nights of cramming for exams in the comfort of your own home. Here are the ins and outs.

Outside

- If you live in a townhouse or freestanding house, make sure that your front door is perfectly visible from the street. Cut back bushes or hedges around your front doors or windows. Eliminate "black holes" in the landscaping to make movements on your property easily visible for police patrolling your neighborhood.
- If there is a fence around your building, you can plant thorny plants such as roses or bougainvillea; this puts an intruder jumping a fence onto your property into a stick-y situation.
- Light up the perimeter by installing motion-sensor lights around the corners of your house.
- Don't put your name on your outdoor mailbox.
- Don't leave an extra key under the mat or in an obvious spot; instead, put an extra key outside, hidden in a secure box with a combination lock.

Inside

- Make sure the landlord has re-keyed the locks since the last tenant moved out.
- Make sure the front door is solid core and has a deadbolt and a peephole.
- Make sure the windows and fire escapes have good locks in working order.
- Install an alarm system with contacts on front and back doors and windows.
- Put your lights on timers when you are away.
- Leave a generic voice-mail greeting on your phone (if you can enlist a man's voice for the recording, even better).
- Make sure that drapes and window blinds are turned so that voyeurs on the outside cannot see in.

Whether you live on or off campus, in a townhouse or a dorm, creating that perimeter of safety allows you to feel safe and secure in your own home. Establishing a good relationship with your roommates and getting things in writing right up front set you up for solid communication and business practices in the future. Who knows, down the road, you might be the one profiled on *MTV Cribs*!

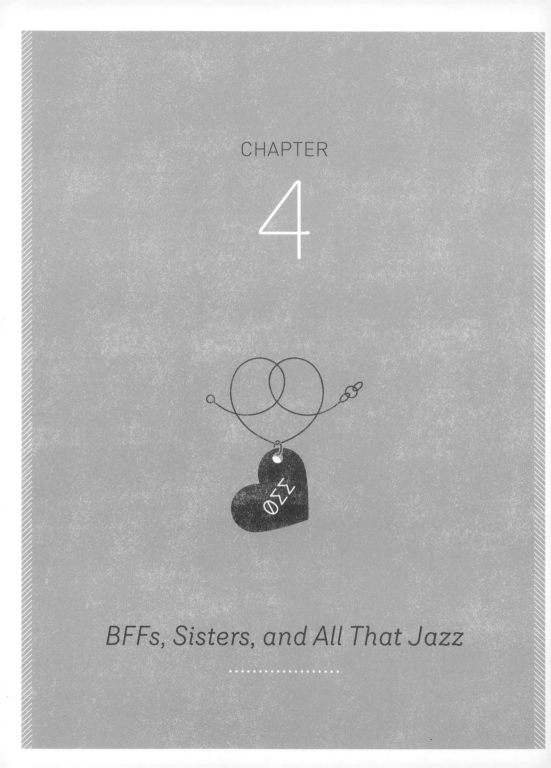

CHAPTER

4

BFFs, Sisters, and All That Jazz

When I was a junior in college, I lived in an apartment off campus. My roommate did not go to UCLA; she was a friend from home who went to Loyola Marymount University a few miles away. I was a member of the Delta Gamma Sorority and a UCLA cheerleader. I was having tons of fun and really enjoying my social life. One night, we had a mixer with a fraternity that was just down the street from my apartment. I met up with a couple of sorority sisters first so I would not have to arrive at the party by myself. We were greeted at the door and some guys handed us plastic cups filled with some sort of punch. As the night wore on, we laughed, mingled, and began to dance. One by one, my sorority sisters hooked up with guys or went off with other friends. I had completely lost track of all of them, because I was out on the dance floor with one of the guys I had just met. That was right about the time that my legs felt like rubber, my shoes were like roller skates, and the whole room started spinning . . .

It turns out the punch had quite a bit of Everclear kick in it—180 proof clear grain alcohol. That's 95 percent alcohol; well over twice as strong as regular alcohols and once listed in the *Guinness Book of World Records* as "the most alcoholic drink." Clearly, our hosts were not fooling around. (See Chapter 5, page 66, to read more about alcohol, drugs, and date abuse.) I suddenly needed help. The nice frat boy who had been giving me the drinks and dancing with me offered to walk me home. I was vaguely coherent at this point and was thankful that someone was able to lead me out of the room. I remember staggering down the front steps of the fraternity, hanging onto the guy's waist. I was able to point and tell him my apartment number. The rest is a blur. When I woke up I was on my bathroom floor; I had apparently gotten sick in the toilet. But what snapped me out of it was my roommate, who was grabbing the nice frat boy by the neck and screaming at him to "get the hell out of our apartment!" You see, he wasn't so nice after all. In fact, he was trying to take off my clothes. Thank God my wonderful roommate intervened.

Let's just think about what kind of guy would want to get it on with a chick who had just puked and was completely out of it! But more importantly, I want to focus on what could have happened, what should have been done differently, and the true meaning of the saying, "A friend in need is a friend indeed."

You have heard it time and time again: "safety in numbers." You see, we sorority sisters should have all stuck together that night. Most of my friends went off to make out with guys or left to go to another party without checking in with everyone else. Let's face it, when you get into the party mode with tons of guys around, music pumping, drinks pouring, it's easy to get distracted and lose sight of where your girlfriends are. I am extremely lucky that I was not raped that night—that, crucially, my brave, strong roommate "had my back."

Understanding and sticking to the Safety Chick Code of Sisterhood (see page 56) could save someone's life, prevent a crime from happening, and help transform insecurities and cattiness into a strong, compassionate, and empowering bond of sisterhood. This chapter will also examine the ways being a college student can lead to self-destructive behavior and show you how to take a breath, relax, and enjoy yourself.

Mean Girls vs. The Sisterhood of the Traveling Pants: A Reality Lesson

Over the years, I have spoken to thousands of young women about personal safety and crime prevention. More importantly, I always try to instill the message that living in a positive and empowered way translates into every aspect of life. When I ask questions about how girls treat each other or how they have helped each other in different situations, I am always amazed that among their stories are many of how mean and hurtful they can be to one another.

Rosalind Wiseman is an incredibly insightful chick—someone I would be proud to have as part of my Safety Chick posse. Rosalind wrote the book *Queen Bees & Wannabes* (Three River Press, 2002), the book that inspired the movie *Mean Girls*.

The movie is about a girl named Cady Heron who grew up in the African bush, home-schooled by her zoologist parents. When Cady and her family have to move back to America and Cady enters public school for the first time, she is greeted by a whole new family of jungle creatures: instead of lions, giraffes, and rhinos, there are jocks, nerds, and the other packs of the high school wilds. She then must learn to deal with the most threatening animal of all—the Queen Bee, aka Regina Jorge, the beautiful, stuck-up, and mean girl who leads the most popular clique. When Cady falls for Regina's boyfriend, jealousy and retaliation take over, making Cady's life very difficult. Regina attempts to destroy Cady's reputation and ruin her social life, until Cady stands up for herself and fights back. Both girls take the term "mean spirited" to a new level.

If you haven't seen it, rent it, because it is the epitome of what I am talking about—and hopefully sinks in the message loud and clear that the catty, backstabbing, social climbing, selfish behavior that is demonstrated in *Mean Girls* is not acceptable, and you should do what you can to stop it when you see it in yourself or others around you. While I am not a psychologist, and have no doctorate degree in psychiatry, I have been a girl/woman for some forty-odd years. I have observed and been a part of the too-many-to-count emotional dramas that accompany women through every stage of growing up. I will be the first to admit that I have been pulled into many a drama, egotistically thinking that I could help in some way. Truth be told, I just became a part of the problem, not the solution.

A counterpart of sorts to *Mean Girls* is a movie called *The Sisterhood of the Traveling Pants*, based on the first book in a series of novels of the same name by Ann Brashares (Delacorte Books, 2003). If you haven't seen it—you guessed it—rent it! It is a wonderful movie that highlights how women can be kind and supportive toward each other. The movie follows four childhood girlfriends through an emotional summer. Faced with going their separate ways after growing up together, the girls find a pair of used jeans in a thrift store that miraculously fits them all perfectly. These "traveling pants" become the symbol of the unbreakable bonds between them, and represent the support of the sisterhood they've found with each other. The pants are also the agent that leads each girl into bruising and ultimately healing confrontations with love and courage. After watching these girls support each other over the years through all the tragedy and triumph and unconditional love, we should all want to strive to have these types of friendships in our own lives. Unlike the vicious undermining and jealous relationships of the teens in *Mean Girls*, these four young women couldn't be closer and genuinely want the best for each other, which, in real life, should be the ultimate goal of any friendship.

The Three Keys of the Safety Chick Code of Sisterhood

As the result of the experiences and ideas from thousands of women I have met over a decade of being the Safety Chick—women of all ages and backgrounds, some crime victims, some never touched by crime, some students, some Soccer Moms—I developed something I call the Code of Sisterhood. I noticed a common theme at every gathering—the women had come to hear me speak because they wanted to be empowered and take safety into their own hands. The keys to the Code are what I believe are missing in many women's lives. You can break the cycle of negative stereotypes and help make our gender into the wonderful, loving, and strong chicks that we were meant to be. Take the steps in your own life to implement the behaviors or thoughts behind these codes. Doing so not only can make you a better friend, it also could help save someone's life.

Communicate

Key #1: Men Are from Mars—But Maybe We Should Visit Their Planet Once in a While

I was raised with two brothers, no sisters. I have been an athlete and around sports my whole life. I even have three boys, no girls. So, needless to say, I have had a lot of opportunity to study men. I have watched as they playfully wrestle with each other one minute, then claw, grab, and punch each other viciously the next. If they get into a disagreement with one of their friends, they might call him every name in the book, they might even threaten to "kick his ass after school"... but there is another thing I always saw: No matter what is said, no matter how loud they yell, after they get it all out and the argument has passed, they are back to being buddies. No hard feeling, no grudges.

Okay, it's a generalization. But often true per those extended observations. Another generalization that bears out: a lot of women don't do that. For some reason, women are often afraid of confrontation or uncomfortable with clearing the air or telling it like it is with each other, perhaps for fear of being thought a bitch or hurting each other's feelings. But women have no problem hanging up the phone on the friend they are fighting with and then calling another friend to complain about it! It kind of pains me to say this, but in these cases, guys are better communicators. Key #1 focuses on how to remedy that. The bottom line is: If you have an issue with one of your girlfriends, take the time to honestly communicate your feelings and urge her to do the same (see the three C's on page 42).

It's Getting Hot in Here
Don't be afraid if your argument gets heated; people are human and sometimes things aren't always copacetic. It is okay to get angry; just don't let things get out of control or off track.

Time Is on Your Side
If the conversation doesn't go according to plan, give your friend and the issues some time; things have a way of sorting themselves out after a while.

Keep It Close to the Vest
Do not bring other people into your disagreement; it just leads to drama and inappropriate gossip.

No Negative = Positive
Do not talk negatively about the girl you are in the argument with just as you would hope she wouldn't be dishing about you.

"I will speak ill of no man and speak all the good I know of everybody."

—Benjamin Franklin

You Get My Back, I'll Get Yours

KEY #2: Chicks Before Dicks

While this phrase is not very elegant, it's a kind of rallying cry that you may hear, if you haven't already, and its meaning for women is meant to be positive and empowering. The saying should be taken as a reminder to help protect each other from sexual predators, abusive boyfriends, and poor safety choices. Think about it: Why is it that a man can wreak havoc on a woman and her friendships? It's a stereotype, but typical enough that when a woman tries to get a guy to change his plans with a buddy or interfere with some sporting event . . . fugeddabout it. Meanwhile, lots of women will drop plans with her friends if a guy calls.

This mindset makes women resentful or jealous of the friend who broke the plans. Most of us have been on the receiving end of friend dumping and it sure doesn't feel good. It perpetuates the feeling of women not trusting each other, the feeling that women don't care about each other, and the feeling that their girlfriends don't have their best interests at heart. The most important thing you can do as a friend is to make sure that you are not one of those "dumpers"—that you respect your friends and the plans that you have committed to; that you have the integrity to communicate honestly and openly if a "guy conflict" should arise. Key #2 is about understanding how to navigate through the world of the opposite sex safely and without hurting your girlfriend relationships in the process.

Friends Don't Let Friends Hook Up

No matter how cute and sexy the person is you just can't trust a stranger. Remind your friend about the handsome and sexy Ted Bundy (the serial killer who lured women into his van and murdered them). Encourage her to get the guy's phone number and call him the next day. Besides, if the guy is worth it, he'll wait.

No Green-Eyed Monsters

Always be supportive of your friends and their relationships. If you have ever had a crush on a guy, you know how euphoric those first few days/weeks/months can be. Don't act jealous or be mean because your buddy hasn't hung out with you as much. On the other hand . . . if you are that girlfriend in love, be sensitive to your friends' feelings, and be sure to carve out some "chick time" as well. Remember: your friends will be there for you long after the crush of the month.

No Sloppy Seconds

There is no worse feeling than breaking up with a guy, and then finding out that your best friend is dating him. Unless it is a very unique situation, that kind of thing is a friendship deal-breaker. Think long and hard before doing something like that. We have all been there; all you have to do is put yourself in your girlfriend's position. Ask yourself, "How would I feel if she did that to me?" If the answer is, *"Horrible!"* then steer clear. A true friend is someone who puts her friends' feelings before her own.

Be Proud, Be Kind, Be Loyal

KEY #3: "Make New Friends but Keep the Old"

That was the title of a song I learned when I was a Camp Fire Girl. We didn't have the good cookies like the Girl Scouts, but we did sell delicious chocolate-mint stick candies! The point is, from a very young age we are taught to cherish our friends, yet somewhere along the way, many people tend to lose sight of the value of friendship. As you get older and life gets more complicated, it's hard to stay in touch with friends, especially when you leave for college. One of the greatest gifts you can give yourself is to make an effort to stay in touch with friends, build new friendships, and always be there for a friend in need. That is at the core of Key #3.

Kiss Me through the Phone

As you leave your home town and most of the friends you know, make an effort to stay connected. In this day of Facebook, Twitter, texting, etc., there is no reason to lose contact with any of your homies. Sometimes, the friends you have known the longest can prove to be the best at helping you navigate through the most difficult or confusing times of your life. Karen Pellizzari Goodman has been my dear friend since kindergarten. Heck—we made our mothers sew us matching outfits to wear to school in fifth grade! We haven't always lived in the same town, we don't have all the same friends, but I know she will always have my back and I will always have hers. That is the gift, the beauty, of cherishing old friendships.

New Friendships Are a Blank Canvas

Enjoy meeting new friends. Be open to meeting people who might be different than you, who might have different hobbies or different cultural backgrounds. Think how boring life would be if everybody were exactly the same—we learn and grow the most by surrounding ourselves with people of different views and interests.

Group Discount

Have fun with all your friends! Encourage women to mingle with each other. Organize events or books clubs that include everybody. The idea is not to create cliques, rather a network of fantastic women of all styles and interests. Embrace rather than alienate!

"My best friend is the one who brings out the best in me." **—Henry Ford**

Taking your friendships seriously should translate into the way you treat all women. Remember: the Safety Chick Code of Sisterhood can save lives. The sooner predators realize that we as women will not put up with their targeting and profiling, the sooner they learn that each of us will be there to help our sister out whether we know her or not, the sooner these cowards will think twice about targeting "defenseless" women.

"A friend is a gift you give yourself." **—Robert Louis Stevenson**

It's All Greek to Me: What to Know about Sororities

The Greek system is a big part of college life. It is filled with wonderful traditions and bonds. Joining a sorority can be an incredible experience, one that creates lifelong friends, but it isn't for everyone and certainly is not a requirement for an amazing college experience. If you do decide to join a house (they call this to "rush"), give it some careful thought and make sure it's a good fit. Here are a few things to consider while you decide if Greek life is right for you.

What to Consider

Group Hug

Do you like being part of a group? It is nice to be a part of a group that is like your family away from home. Whether you live in the sorority house or not, you will have a place to go where you can curl up on the couch with your "sisters" to unwind, chat, and feel supported.

Susie Social

Are you someone who loves to plan, organize, fund-raise, create? Sororities have tons of activities and events to participate in and be a part of.

Tight Budget

Sororities have dues and other expenses that can be costly, so be sure to ask how much all the fees are. Ask a member what she typically spends a year on sorority stuff.

Rush and Rejection

There is a weeklong evaluation process you must go through to join a sorority. This is a chance for the different groups to meet you, and for you to get acquainted with the different houses and their members. In addition, it is an opportunity for them to evaluate you to see if you would be a good fit for their group, and a time for you to see if they are right for you. Be prepared for the sting of rejection if the house you want to be in does not choose you. If this process sounds miserable to you, you shouldn't do it. And if you don't get your first choice, oftentimes your second choice was where you fit in the best in the first place (if you know what I mean).

As with any commitment to community and every family, membership in a sorority includes responsibilities for being conscientious and taking care of yourself. There are certain times or situations throughout your sorority life, should you choose to join, that you could encounter some safety issues. The key is to always make smart personal-safety choices and with your sisters, always have each others' back. With that said, it is important to be aware of an activity known as "hazing."

Hazing

You have probably heard of hazing, and it's a troubling topic indeed. Descending from the tradition of rites of passage, hazing has often been a common part of initiating new members into fraternities and sororities. The phenomenon takes to an extreme the theory that testing the endurance of new members of a group through an ordeal of shared suffering will promote group loyalty—often an irresponsible extreme, and the practices have been in recent decades subject to much controversy and new controls.

According to HazingPrevention.org, hazing is any action taken or situation created intentionally to embarrass, ridicule, intimidate, or humiliate members of a group or team, or cause physical or emotional harm. The definition includes both new and current members of the group, and counts whether participation is forced or the person is willing. While there may be forms of hazing that are benign or even good-humored, reckless or punishing rituals are still being carried out. Again according to HazingPrevention.org, hazing is simply organized bullying. The consequences of students who participate in hazing are becoming quite severe. Recently six sorority girls at a major university were arrested and charged with felony hazing. Not only were they expelled from school, but they will now face criminal penalties and possible prison time.

If you are thinking of becoming part of a sorority, you need to know how to protect yourself from hazing and what your rights and options are. Hazing often includes binge drinking (see Chapter 5, page 66), a very dangerous undertaking that can lead to other kinds of grave physical danger, including sexual abuse. Read the following sections carefully to help you recognize when the fun part of joining turns into something inappropriate.

Once you are invited to join a particular sorority, you are given a "bid." If you decide that this is the house you want to join, you then become a "pledge." The "pledge period" is a time when you interact more with the group and get to know your sisters better. During this time, you'll learn more about the traditions and history of the sorority as well as the commitments and events you will be required to attend. Once this pledge period is over, you participate in an initiation ceremony that makes you an official "sister" of the sorority. Pledge period is also the most common time for hazing to occur.

If you feel that you are a victim of hazing, or if someone is trying to get you to participate, here are some things that you can do:

Don't Isolate

Be aware if someone or a group is trying to keep you away from your friends outside the group. Many hazers attempt to keep their victims from people who might challenge or question them.

No Secrets

Many people who abuse demand secrecy either through threats or intimidation. You have a right to tell anyone anything about what is going on. Talk with others either in your group or outside about what is happening.

Power in Numbers

Get together with other people in the group who are being hazed and band together and refuse to be hazed. There is always safety and power in numbers.

Walk Away

I know this might be hard to do, but you ALWAYS have the right to quit the group. Besides, who wants to belong to an organization that would abuse its members or so-called "sisters"?

If you find yourself in a situation as a pledge that makes you at all uncomfortable, and initial talks or banding with your fellow pledges to protest does not alleviate it, do not hesitate to seek guidance from your parents, a counselor, or a school official. Being a sister in a sorority should be a wonderful, bonding experience. If you know of hazing going on at your school, report it. Don't let a few bad apples spoil the bunch.

Don't Worry; Be Happy: How to Cope with Stress

Making the jump from high school to college can mean a much more intense workload. Combine that with your newfound freedom and social life, and things can get a little out of control. Learning how to deal with stress and developing time-management skills can make your college experience much more enjoyable. The first year, you might want to take things slowly—get used to your new academic schedule, and assess how much time is needed to get all your work done BEFORE you start volunteering to be the co-chair of the Luau Party at your sorority or the social director of your dorm. Take it easy on yourself. Don't set unreal expectations. Taking all advanced upper grad classes as a freshman and expecting to get all A's in addition to working full time at the student bookstore might be a bit overzealous. Talk with your counselor about your overall schedule and come up with a realistic balance of school and work. Other factors cause stress as well—parental pressures, homesickness, finances. Talk to your parents and roommates so they can help you deal with any stress you may be experiencing.

The Physical Toll of Stress

New findings on the effects of stress are sobering and alarming. Stress can be brutal both mentally and physically. It has been linked to headaches, heartburn, sudden variations in weight, and other more harmful symptoms like ulcers and cardiovascular disorders. Stress can also cripple you emotionally; it can translate into a recurring feeling of hopelessness in coping with life. Stress sufferers can burst suddenly into tears or, even worse—when overcome with sadness find themselves unable to cry.

Geez! These are not the ingredients for a favorable quality of life—definitely not a part of the Safety Chick lifestyle. So, in the words of that cute singer Jesse McCartney in his song "Leavin'": "Don't stress, don't stress, don't stress." Following are some straightforward tools for coping, all of them simple to employ and really easy to forget in the whirlwind of school life—but crucial to your mental and physical health.

Take the Time to Realize You Are Stressed

That might sound funny, but when you are in the middle of your daily life, running from point A to point B, you might not be aware that you are stressed out. If you are feeling overwhelmed or out of sorts, be honest with yourself and admit that you are stressed. Once you do that, you can take steps to deal with things. Living in denial only makes matters worse and prolongs your misery!

Get Some ZZZ's

Do not forget or underestimate the importance of a good night's sleep! If you are burning the candle at both ends, it will catch up with you. Make a conscious effort to forgo a party or an extra study session to get a few more hours of sleep. Getting some solid shut-eye can help you feel refreshed and recharged, and help you see things more clearly in the morning.

The 2006 Sleep in America poll by the National Sleep Foundation showed that 80 percent of teens don't get the recommended amount of sleep. At least 28 percent fall asleep in school and 22 percent fall asleep doing homework.

Put Some Healthy Fuel in Your Body

Have your healthy eating habits fallen by the wayside because of your busy schedule? Do you find yourself grabbing fast food or whatever is in the vending machines on a regular basis? Remember: You truly are what you eat. Getting some fruits, veggies, grains, and proteins into your system really is essential to a balanced diet—a legendary concept in itself that is also absolutely true for your well-being—and could be just the thing to get you back when you've fallen off track. And no, jalapeño-flavored potato chips don't count as a vegetable.

Let's Get Physical

Whether you work out on a regular basis or not, even a little exercise is better than nothing—get out, take a walk, clear your head. Getting your blood pumping and working up a sweat is good for the heart and the soul.

Laugh Out Loud

It also really helps to develop a good sense of humor. As you live and grow, it is amazing how laughter gets you through even the toughest times. Learning to laugh at yourself keeps things in perspective—it reminds you to not be so hard on yourself. Laughing also releases endorphins, which help with happy thoughts.

Try to make these stress-reducing tactics a part of your daily regime, and reach for them to help when you are feeling inundated or down. If your feelings become too overwhelming, seek help promptly from a professional. There are people specifically charged with helping you in a wide range of situations that may come up, and there is no shame or embarrassment in going to them for help with stress. The campus women's health center is a great place to start for more assistance.

Women, Body Image, and Being Perfect

What the media and our society have created with regard to women's body image drives me crazy. While we all know that realistically there is no such thing as a "perfect body," subconsciously a lot of us struggle with what is real versus what is ideal and spend way too much time focusing on our appearance.

In college, living with a group of women in a dorm or sorority house can sometimes magnify this fixation on how we look. It can be so much fun getting ready to go out with your roommates, all sharing one bathroom—deciding what to wear, what color eye shadow to put on, etc. Putting ourselves together is a great part of being female. But being surrounded by talk about being fat or skinny, tall or short, pretty or not, can make some women obsess a little too much. For some, if the obsession gets out of control, it can create an eating disorder. Eating disorders are serious illnesses and can be life-threatening. If you or someone you know has an eating disorder, act immediately to nip it in the bud. There are many wonderful organizations out there to help you. See the Resources section on page 192.

Building strong friendships, building skills for coping with difficult situations, and keeping a healthy mind and body all work together to create a lifestyle that is productive and positive. Enjoy all the trials and tribulations that college life has to offer, and make lifelong friends in the process.

Safety Chick Checklist:
Five Ways to Reduce Stress

JUST CHILL | Make some alone time for yourself. Take a break from the hectic schedule and crazy pace. Find a quiet space—in the corner of the library with the sun gently warming you through the windowpanes or on a serene park bench. Allowing yourself some private time to just sit and chill helps clear the cobwebs and organize your thoughts.

PRINCESS FOR A DAY | If you feel run down and neglected, a quick trip to the spa for a massage or the nail salon for a mani-pedi can do just the trick! If money is tight, why don't you and your friends have a "Beauty Night" complete with refreshments and facials and mud packs from the local drug store. Sometimes just a little pampering is all you need to feel refreshed.

GET YOUR GROOVE ON | There is no better way to release pent-up energy than exercise. If running or kickboxing isn't your thing, try dancing your stress away. Crank your iTunes and shake your booty around your room—just make sure your shades are drawn (lol).

GLASS HALF FULL | Stress can really be mind over matter. Make the decision to focus on the positive. A happy, constructive mindset can truly make a difference in your overall well-being.

THE WHOLE ENCHILADA | When your mind feels full to bursting with stress, take your focus off the little things like your statistics quiz tomorrow or the parking ticket you got at lunch. Instead, nudge yourself to step back and think about the big picture. Heck—do you even remember what you had for dinner last Wednesday? Was it Mexican food? Likewise, that embarrassing thing you said to that guy or the paper you turned in that you weren't happy with. Don't sweat the small stuff. Learning how to put things in perspective comes from remembering that "this too shall pass."

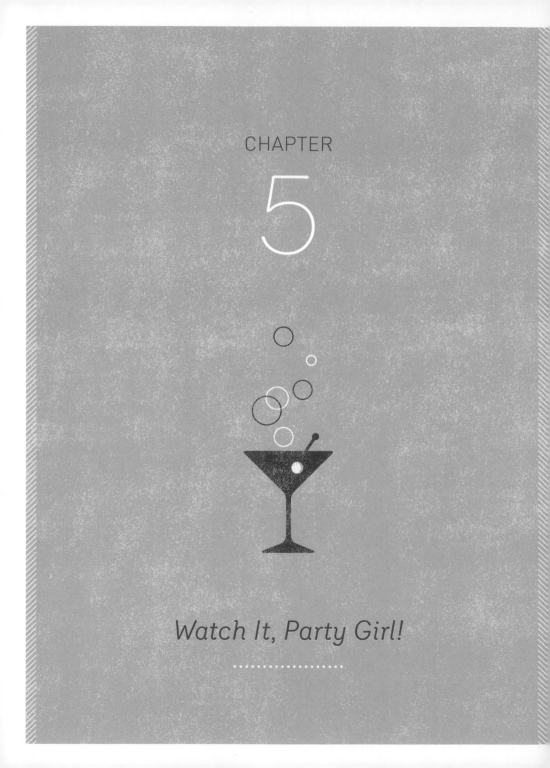

CHAPTER

5

Watch It, Party Girl!

A young woman was in her first year at a well-respected Ivy League college. In a date rape discussion group, she told of how she'd had a false sense of security because of the clean-cut and safe ethos that her school and student body was known for.

She had gone to her winter formal with a guy she considered her best friend. She said he seemed like one of those classic nice guys— always there to help with dating problems, brought her soup when she was sick, etc. When he picked her up for the dance that night, he brought her flowers, and then took her to a nice dinner—as "just friends." She even remarked on how polite he was, opening the car door for her, telling her how great she looked—a total gentleman.

After the dance, he invited her back to his room where, he said, he had a surprise waiting: he had decorated his room with balloons and flowers. He even had a bottle of champagne on ice. Normally she did not drink, but she felt very comfortable with her friend. Sharing a bit of champagne seemed harmless enough—it was, after all, a big night, and she was in a "safe" environment. It was the wee hours of the morning. She sipped her champagne, and suddenly, immediately, she became really tired. Minutes later, she passed out on his couch. When she woke up, her "friend" was having sex with her.

There are countless stories like this one, about students getting hurt from alcohol- or drug-related incidents while partying. While some of the best memories you will make in college will happen at parties, football games, sorority or fraternity functions, dances, and other social events, any or all of these may include people drinking alcohol or using drugs. Perhaps ironically, partying is serious business: consider the risks involved with using substances that affect your body and impair your judgment. Your responsibilities are huge if you choose to use them or be around other people who are. The tricky thing is, loosening up your sense of responsibility is *exactly* what drugs and alcohol are used for, or at least a big part of their appeal. It is vital that you understand the effects of these substances and how to navigate the safety challenges of parties before entering this arena. This chapter will cover basic party safety, the dangers of binge drinking, what experts now categorize as Drug Facilitated Sexual Assault (DFSA), what so-called date rape drugs are, and what to do if you or a friend has been raped.

Binge Drinking

Binge drinking is the consumption of excessive amounts of alcohol in a short period of time. An article written by Leslie Thompson on www.collegebingedrinking.com states that nearly 44 percent of college students are binge drinkers, which means 2 out of 5 students regularly consume 4 or 5 alcoholic drinks within a two-hour period.

Whether you drink or not, there most likely will be times in your college career that you will find yourself in a binge-drinking situation: frat parties, formals, tailgates, dorm functions, etc. So it is best to know the facts and really understand the danger before something tragic happens. One of my dear friends lost her handsome, gregarious, college baseball star to binge drinking and I have witnessed the excruciating pain his family and friends still endure to this day. One of the reasons binge-drinking deaths are so tragic is because they are senseless and preventable.

Look—I am not trying to be unrealistic and suggest that you will never be a part of social drinking. What I am saying is that the responsibility is on YOU to know your limits and stay within them. Alcohol has a way of sneaking up on you. You can be fine one moment and very, very drunk the next. That is why it is important to always go with a buddy to parties where there is going to be alcohol; keep your girlfriends close and be very aware of what and how much you are drinking.

Don't think binge drinking is just for frat boys or football players. The Society for Women's Health Research (SWHR) Web site posted startling results from a study that showed the percentage of women drinkers has drastically increased over the last fifteen years or so. The results were from the Harvard School of Public Health College Alcohol Study, which was set up to examine drinking behavior among men and women in college. In addition, female students who fell into the category of "frequent binge drinkers" jumped from 5 to 12 percent among women at all women's colleges. The number increased at coed colleges, as well.

Do yourself a favor: Know your limits with alcohol—and make that determination when you are sober, not drunk. If you're going to drink, be safe and make SMART personal safety choices:

- Do not drink to excess.
- Beware of shots! If you're in a situation where drinking seems to be getting out of control, do not get drawn in—just say "No!" to doing shots and chugging drinks. This will help you stay alert.
- Beware of being "over-served." Yes, it is absolutely your responsibility to know your drinking limits. But sometimes there are people doing their very best—let's say in the innocent but heedless spirit of the party—to make you overindulge, and that can lead you past your best judgment or make you afraid to refuse. Do not be! It's always okay to acknowledge that you have had too much to drink and need to go home. Have a trusted friend give you a ride home and tuck you safely into bed.
- Do not isolate yourself or leave alone if you feel drunk. Seek out help and a safe place at once.
- Help any student who appears to be dangerously intoxicated.
- Do not leave an intoxicated person you are assisting by herself. Get help, and call 911.

Read the rest of this chapter carefully to arm yourself for some of the biggest and most important challenges to your safety at college.

DFSA (Drug Facilitated Sexual Assault) Happens

A while back, when I was doing research for an episode of *America's Most Wanted* (more on that below), I met a woman who is the leading expert in "drug facilitated sexual assault." Her name is Trinka Porrata, and she is one amazing Safety Chick herself! She, along with the Shortridges, (who lost their son to a GHB overdose), started the organization Project GHB, named for one of the most commonly used of the disorienting or severely incapacitating drugs now typically referred to as date rape drugs—so called because they are used by people who exploit their access or right to belong in a normal social situation. The predator effectively sneaks "poison" into another person's drink so that person may yield to physical demands from the predator, or simply be too incapacitated to be conscious of what is happening. Trinka has made it her mission to educate law enforcement officials, the media, and the general public about this horrific crime and the drugs that go along with it. She has been extremely helpful to me over the years and educated me on all of her hard-won research to help spread the word about these drugs and the predators who use them, some of which I'm sharing with you here.

According to Trinka, DFSA has traditionally been defined as Drug Facilitated Sexual Assault by use of an anesthesia-type drug (whether taken voluntarily or given surreptitiously by a suspect), rendering the victim physically incapacitated or otherwise unable to give or withhold consent. Current interpretation also considers the use of a wider scope of drugs, not just depressants. At a rough count, more than forty drugs have been utilized in this manner. Trinka says most provide at least some degree of amnesia, disinhibition, and in some cases outright loss of consciousness, minimizing the victim's ability to resist, protect herself/himself, or recount details of events. (I'll get into the specifics of these drugs a bit later on.)

Many of these drugs are not routinely included in drug testing by hospital and police labs, and are thus easily overlooked, especially when training on DFSA issues is limited or absent. Some of the drugs leave the victim's system so quickly, it is unlikely a positive toxicology report will be possible in most cases.

Anyone can be a victim of this crime. Drug rape victims come in all ages and sizes and from all ethnic, cultural, and economic backgrounds. It may be a student; it can also be an instructor or a staff member or support personnel. It can be ANYONE. And, yes, it can happen to men as well as women.

Here are Trinka's thoughts on the reality of date-rape drugs:

For starters, let's forget the term that's heard so often in the media: "date-rape drug." Drugs neither know nor care whether or not someone is on a date. Let's talk about "rape drugs" or "predatory drugs." There are at least forty of them, starting with alcohol and running throughout the drug alphabet. "Rape drugs" are substances used to facilitate a sexual assault. Their effects vary but the end result is the same—the person is rendered unable to knowingly give or withhold consent to a sexual act and typically remembers little or nothing about it. In fact, the person may not even know who committed the assault. These drugs work all too well, so prevention is the first choice, followed by immediate and thorough investigation, and meaningful resolution.

Silence Is Not Golden

It is difficult to measure silence, but it is estimated that more than half of all sexual assaults go unreported. This may be particularly true with drug rapes, as the lack of knowledge of what happened makes it even more difficult to report the incident. Amnesia can't be proven, increasing the victim's fear of his or her story not being believed. Unfortunately, the experiences of some who have come forward support that fear—their stories were dismissed, disbelieved, or reclassified. Evidence is often not taken or delayed too long, even when the victim has come forward.

According to Campus Crime Stats at www.securityoncampus.org, "Fewer than 5 percent of completed and attempted rapes were reported to law enforcement officials. In about two-thirds of the campus rape incidents, however, the victim did tell another person about the incidents."

Within the stats for reporting of all rapes, there are simply no solid statistics regarding the number of drug rapes. Separate statistics are not maintained by most law enforcement agencies. In addition, testing issues and lack of awareness make it difficult to accurately identify drug rapes.

A True (and All Too Common) Story

Over the years, Trinka Porrata (see page 69) has come across hundreds of victims and the tragic stories that go with them—here is a very powerful one.

At a West Coast university, a female student went with others to a large fraternity party. She had a few beers; the last one was given to her already opened. Her friends noticed that she suddenly became quite drunk. They had never seen her that way. During this time, a star football player had been coming on to her (someone her friends knew was of no interest to her), and a friend moved her away from him at one point. Her friends decided to take her back to the sorority house and drove her there. She got out of the car and headed, staggering, toward the house as her friends drove away.

She woke up the next day with a headache and stomach pains. She had no memory of leaving the party, of her friends taking her home, or anything thereafter. Her bra and tube top were around her waist; her pants were on the floor. Her body was dirt stained, and on the chair was a jacket belonging to the football player. The jacket had dirt and blood on it. Her underwear was missing.

She was scared and confused. Friends were also disturbed by her condition. Rumors immediately began to fly. Word was that the football star was bragging that he had had sex with her in the dirt outside the sorority house. He was also bragging about being in possession of her underwear. She was known to her friends to be a virgin and she was proud of that, although it also meant she had to take some teasing about it. Her friends knew that she would not have chosen to have a first sexual experience with that man, and definitely not that way.

E-mails, phone calls, and conversations began to flow between male and female students about the incident. The suspect's closest friend immediately began making calls to girls who knew the victim, telling them that she was a liar and calling her derogatory names. Meanwhile, the victim went to the hospital and reported the incident to police. The victim stated that she had consumed more beer on previous occasions without experiencing anything similar in terms of loss of memory, illness, etc. The assigned detective conducted an exhaustive investigation with detailed interviews of every possible witness. The suspect's best friend systematically tried to discredit the victim in his police interview by describing her as a slut who flirted and allowed anyone to fondle her and drank a lot—testimony that was inconsistent with the other witnesses'. But even he described the sexual conduct of the suspect with the victim in detail, and thereby inadvertently laid out damning evidence. He described the victim as having been "too drunk to know what was happening," which would mean that the suspect *knew* she was unable to give or withhold consent.

But ultimately the prosecutor's office issued an announcement declining prosecution. The statement claimed that there was "insufficient evidence to meet the statutory elements of rape of any degree." The detective was rightfully livid. It appeared that the prosecutor's office had bowed to the threats made by the university (documented calls from the university's attorney to the prosecutor's office). After all, this was their star football player, and that was the most important factor in the end. The prosecutor's statement had claimed that since the victim couldn't remember, there was no proof that she hadn't given consent. He cited the need to prove that the victim was either "physically helpless or mentally incapable of consent." The statement said there was no evidence to support that she was "unconscious or for any other reason physically unable to communicate unwillingness to act." And, it said, there was no evidence that she was mentally incapacitated, meaning she was unable to "understand the nature or consequences of the act of sexual intercourse whether that condition is produced by illness, defect, the influence of a substance or from some other cause." Stunning, given the detailed account numerous witnesses gave of her dramatic change to being suddenly very intoxicated, and her inability to stand or walk normally on her own.

The decision was even more shocking in the light of another, independent witness: This person who called police during the very night of the incident, to report a possible rape in progress on the campus—right beside that sorority house. The witness was walking home; he had not been drinking that night. As he passed the location he observed a female leaning against the wall, arms at her side, with a male standing in front of her. He said that he looked right at her, and she looked like there was "no one home. Her eyes were glazed, like she was drugged." She made no effort to cover herself as he passed, he said, though she was wearing only a bra and maybe underwear. He said she looked "really out of it," and it didn't seem right to him. The male then pulled her around the corner, out of his view. His account clearly matched the time and descriptions of the victim and the football player. When police arrived, they were gone. In the end, a suspect openly bragged about his sexual escapades, waved his victim's panties for all to see, and walked away from criminal prosecution. A tragic story, and hardly a way to provide an aura of safety for female students. But most of all, a grim reminder of why YOU have to take care of YOURSELF.

Where Does DFSA Happen?

Understanding the situations and locations where DFSA's are likely to occur can help you assess and make determinations on how and where you want to socialize. Remember—the more you know, the better decisions you will make when it comes to your safety.

Parties

As I have emphasized throughout these pages, while college offers new levels of freedom, those freedoms come with new responsibilities, new stress factors, peer pressure, and increased exposure to social relationships, drugs, and sex. Freshmen are especially vulnerable and less well equipped for these new challenges because so much is going on and everything is new at once. In the swirl, it can be tempting to experiment with drugs and/or excessive drinking. But what starts as a choice can result in an intoxicated state with lost control and vulnerability to sexual assault or other forms of abuse (being photographed in compromising positions, robbed, etc.). Remember, even if the act of taking a drink or drug was voluntary, it NEVER constitutes consent to sexual relations.

Granted, letting loose by using substances does complicate the issues of public attitude. Opinion of others in the community, as well as potential jurors and judges, for example, often goes against a person who has behaved in this fashion. This goes a long way in explaining why, when loss of control results in a rape or other abuse, many victims do not report the crime. This is something to think hard about when considering your right to party versus your responsibility for your own safety.

Drinking from the punch bowl at a fraternity party, for example, may be high risk. As one young man put it, "Why don't the girls get it? They drink from the punch bowl, but the guys aren't. Duh, it's laced with more alcohol than they realize or DRUGS. Then they wonder why they wake up naked in some bedroom in the frat house. They HOPE it was the cute guy they were talking to at the punch bowl but it was really one guy and then another and then another . . . sad stuff." Shocked, ashamed, and unsure of what really transpired, the victim may not bother to report the situation at all. Or, she may report it, only to be told in essence, "That's what you get for going to parties like that." Blaming the victim is all too common.

Nightclubs

Nightclubs and bars used by the campus community, while seemingly more secure than student parties, are another prime risk site for DFSA. Put all the rules of making yourself DFSA safe at parties in the previous section to use. On top of that, be aware that nightclubs have special powers to seduce or confuse. The simple fact of loud, professionally pumped music can be disorienting or create adrenaline. Then there's the fact that bars are in the business of selling drinks, and stirring up exhibitionism can be a great way to keep things flowing.

Now, here's a fact that may be surprising but is very important: the first line of opportunity to dose a drink is the bartender. Yes, it does happen. It is particularly likely in clubs catering to students, holding wet T-shirt contests and openly allowing drinking contests. In one Florida incident, the bartender befriended a young lady too shy to enter the wet T-shirt contest, offered a drink on the house, and drugged her. She nearly died that night and the bar was busted for having GHB "on tap." Horrifyingly, they were manufacturing GHB in the basement, had a line running to the bar, and could routinely serve a dose to patrons, willing or not.

You may be thinking, "People are sometimes *willing*?" Sometimes. That is, sometimes young women, for a lot of reasons—some of them strange and complicated, some of them spontaneous—plunge willingly into risky and risqué behavior, drinking or doing drugs, or aspiring to be on *Girls Gone Wild*. Or all of the above. But not all of those girls had any idea what they were doing. Many of the predatory DFSA drugs loosen a person's inhibitions and some, such as GHB, can actually stimulate sexual conduct that is completely out of character for the person. Needless to say, spring break activities are classic opportunities for drug rapes to occur. (See Chapter 7, page 112, for more about spring break.)

It Doesn't Just Happen at the Disco

Sexual assault can happen any time or place. As discussed above, parties and clubs, where drinking is seemingly inevitable, are common grounds but any event where food and drink are being consumed is an opportunity for drugging to occur, since ingestion in some form is typically necessary. Remember: this information is to keep you aware of the dangers, not to scare you into staying at home and ordering delivery pizza every night.

There have been incidents reported where nothing was ingested but victims had tanning cream or massage cream rubbed on them, resulting in blackout periods and sexual assault. The disabling substance may have been in the creams, possibly added by a penetrating substance such as DMSO solvent. Don't take lotion from a stranger. 'Nuff' said.

Drugging may occur at one location and the assault elsewhere, yet the victim may not have knowingly gone with the suspect. A victim may recall getting sleepy and curling up on a couch but then waking up on another couch or bed. Often this change is explained away by the suspect saying simply that he or "they" moved her there to be more comfortable, to be away from the noise, etc. Do NOT let your guard down just because an event seems to be less about partying; you still need to keep your safety radar on.

How Does DFSA Happen?

A few years ago, I hosted a segment for *America's Most Wanted* on date rape drugs. I wanted to show viewers how the predator gets the drug into his victim's drink. We hired three young male actors, and had young women come to what they thought was an audition for a show on dating. We placed hidden cameras strategically throughout the bar. We filled the bar with extras and I watched from a control room above the bar on video monitors. I instructed the male actors to "drug" the girls' drinks whenever they left them unattended.

The most common date rape drugs are gamma hydroxy butyrate (GHB) and Rohypnol. They are both clear substances that look like water. The predators usually disguise the drug by pouring it into small repurposed bottles from things like breath drops, nasal drops, or eye drops. A few drops is all it takes to render a victim helpless. A victim of these drugs can go very quickly from feeling fine to feeling very dizzy, cloudy, and nauseous. A few seconds later she can become extremely disoriented, and therefore very vulnerable. In the worst, most tragic cases, they can die.

For our experiment, we filled dropper bottles with water and the guys wore button cameras so the audience could watch the whole thing through the eyes of the "predator." It was amazing to see how easy it was for these guys to dose the girls' drinks. Most of the young women put their drinks down to go to the bathroom, play pool, and other ordinary reasons. Another common technique: the guy would go to the bar to get a drink for the unsuspecting girl, then simply drug it on the way back to the table. At the end of the segment, we came clean to the young women and told them about the experiment. Every girl was shocked and shaken at how easy it was for the guys to drug their drinks.

What Does a Drug Rapist Look Like?

Bad guys come in a wide spectrum in terms of age, size, and appearance and ethnic, cultural, and economic backgrounds. The drug rapist may be the inarticulate recluse who finds establishing relationships difficult at any level. He may be a stranger or acquaintance lurking in the shadows across the room, just waiting for his target to leave her drink or food unattended to give him a chance to dose it. He may be the unobtrusive figure next to his victim at the bar or table, just quietly reaching past his target for a napkin or pretzel (with a little vial of his drug of choice in the palm of his hand, ready for a quick squeeze into the drink as he reaches beyond it). But the drug rapist may also be the most likable, articulate, suave guy in town. He could be the victim's best friend, or a new acquaintance *trying* to be the best friend, for the moment. He could be that buff guy at the gym or within a campus sports program, patiently showing his target how to use the gym equipment and enticing him or her into trying a new "energy tonic" to help with workout strength or sleep. Ultimately, a druggist may not look like the typical strung-out guy who loiters on the street corner; as with most criminals, they come in all shapes and sizes.

Why Does DFSA Happen?

Sexual assault isn't necessarily about sex. It is often really about power. Drugging someone truly takes power away from her in ways that make being caught and prosecuted even more difficult.

Convicted drug rapist Andrew Luster (a notorious case because of his status as an heir to the Max Factor cosmetics fortune) was articulate and sociable. Some of his victims had actually had consensual sex with him. But part of his sexual pleasure involved having power over unconscious females, as described chillingly, in his own voice, in videotapes of his assaults shown to the jury. Luster is now serving 124 years in prison.

The Most Common Drugs Used in Sexual Assault

I think it is important to name and explain the most common date rape drugs that are out there and their effects. The data that follows was obtained at the time of publication from the Drug Enforcement Agency of the Department of Justice. If you have questions or want to know about other types of drugs, refer to the Resources chapter at the end of the book.

Alcohol is still number one in the sexual assault world. It is involved in some capacity in the majority of sexual assaults. This is in part simply a reflection of the fact that alcohol is a common factor in social events. The fact that alcohol was consumed does not constitute a drug rape. Drug rape can result from voluntary consumption of excessive alcohol, becoming incapable of giving or withholding consent, and then being taken advantage of by a suspect. Voluntary intoxication is risky behavior but it is not in itself blanket consent for anyone to have sex with that person. Accidental consumption of excessive alcohol (drinks being made with double shots or vodka being added since it is relatively tasteless and the drinker unaware of the content or amount, or drugs added surreptitiously) may also result in a person becoming overly intoxicated and then being assaulted. Unfortunately, a high blood alcohol level is often met with criticism and blame directed at the victim. Rapists have been known to employ a drug to disable the victim and then feed her additional alcohol, knowing that the high level will discredit the victim when she swears, "but I only had two drinks!" The blood alcohol level is used to show that the victim is lying when in fact the person may be simply reporting the amount that she willingly and knowingly consumed.

Barbiturates such as sleeping pills, muscle relaxants, motion sickness medications, antihistamines, cold medicines, and pain medications also cause effects that would facilitate sexual assault, especially if mixed with alcohol. The sleeping pill Ambien has been identified in a number of drug rapes, as well as other sleeping pills. Diphenhydramine (an ingredient in cold medications such as Benadryl) has also been reportedly used in a number of rape cases; this drug makes one groggy and sleepy, especially when mixed with alcohol. A wide array of these drugs has been found in toxicology results in rape cases.

Benzodiazepine drugs such as alprazolam (Xanax), clonazepam (Klonopin or Rivotril), chlordiazepoxide (Librium), diazepam (Valium), flunitrazepam (Rohypnol, aka "roofies"), flurazepam (Dalmane), lorazepam (Ativan), and triazolam (Halcion) are frequently used by predators because they are also commonly prescribed around the world. If a victim is taking a prescribed benzodiazepine, the interaction with alcohol, or any other drug added by a predator, could result in incapacitation. Flunitrazepam, often referred to as "roofies," is most commonly cited in the media as a date rape drug, but in reality this drug is not approved for medical use in the United States and is thus far less available than the other benzodiazepine drugs. All of these drugs qualify as rape drugs and all have shown up in toxicology results in rape investigations. Some of these drugs, however, do not show up well, if at all, in drug-screening tests. A confirmation test should be done if the symptoms and timing indicate a possible benzo drug was involved.

Chloral hydrate is the drug that was the original "Mickey Finn" decades ago. The term "slipped a Mickey" is now commonly used to refer to any drug being given someone to knock her out or to cause lack of control and/or loss of memory.

Gamma hydroxy butyrate, or GHB, is one of the most dangerous drugs used as a weapon of rape and is also one of the most difficult to detect because of its rapid metabolism in the body and because not all medical and law enforcement agencies are adequately aware of how to test for it. GHB can cause rapid, dramatic, and bizarre conduct followed by amnesia. It can also cause dangerous depression of respiration, profound coma, and even death. Vomiting, loss of control of body functions, and seizurelike activity are also common side effects. Someone who has overdosed on GHB may slip into unarousable sleep or coma with dramatic snoring activity. Protecting her airway is crucial; she should be kept on her left side, and should NOT be left unattended face down or on her back. GHB overdose can cancel a victim's protective gag reflex, making her at risk of literally drowning in her own vomit. In the campus scene, particular attention should be paid to the possibility of GHB being involved if the allegation involves school athletes or anyone whose body build indicates regular gym use, as GHB and steroids go hand in hand. GHB rapists are often GHB users, and GHB is available in some gyms disguised as muscle-enhancement products.

Ketamine is primarily used as a small-animal tranquilizer for surgical procedures. It can produce a "frozen" state in which the person may feel no pain and become immobile and thus unable to protect herself from assault. It can also produce hallucinations and frightening flashbacks. Though ketamine is often hyped as one of the top date rape drugs, in reality rapists don't use it widely. Other animal tranquilizers have also been used to facilitate rape.

Illegal drugs such as marijuana, heroin, MDMA (Ecstasy) and related hallucinogens, LSD, and mushrooms can cause sedation that can also result in drug rape. Voluntary consumption of illicit drugs puts one at higher risk of such incidents. Thus, one way to prevent assault is to avoid drug use. Unfortunately, rape victims are often afraid to report promptly, fearing positive toxicology tests will expose their voluntary drug use. But voluntary drug usage, even of illicit drugs, does not negate rape. The important thing is for the assault victim to be up front about it and let the detective and prosecutor handle it. The rapist may also give these drugs surreptitiously to cause desired effects or simply to confuse the victim or the police; it works all too well at causing chaos. While many of these drugs (MDMA and hallucinogens) cause stimulation rather than sedation, they are considered rape drugs because while under the influence the person may not be able to make judgment calls. Including hallucinogens as predatory drugs is a relatively new concept but is widely accepted by drug rape experts.

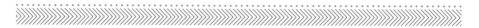

How to Prevent DFSA

Now that I have explained, with the help of Trinka's expertise, the whats, wheres, and whys of DFSA, it is vital that you follow these Safety Chick Tips for how to keep yourself, and your drink, safe.

Drink Responsibly

TIP #1 IF YOU NEED TO POWDER YOUR NOSE, SO DOES YOUR DRINK

- Always know where your beverage came from and don't let it out of your sight.

Never Leave Your Drink Unattended
If you have to use the restroom bring your drink; if you hit the dance floor, bring your drink; if you are immersed in conversation, hold your drink; if you have to make a phone call, take your drink. (Get the idea?) Don't rely on your friends to watch your beverage. All it takes is one distraction (a cute guy walking by, for example) for someone to sneak the drug into your drink. If you realize you slipped and left your drink unattended even for a short time, don't take the chance— throw it away and get a new one.

Never Accept a Drink from a Stranger
Beware of a stranger walking up to you at a party or club and handing you a drink. If possible, restrict your party refreshments to a beverage that you can open yourself (e.g., bottled water, soda, or beer). If you did not see a drink being poured, or if it is ready to serve but in an open container, jettison it.

Never Drink Out of an Open Punch Bowl
Spiking a punch bowl used to mean sneaking in a flask of your parents' alcohol to the school dance. It now takes on a whole new meaning. Opt for the sealed beverage and skip the punch.

Don't Drink Out of a Container That Is Being Passed Around
I must be getting old, because just the thought of this grosses me out! Despite the obvious germs that can be exchanged, you never know what has been slipped into the beverage.

If Your Drink Tastes Funny, Get Rid of It
If your drink has been tainted, it might taste salty or have unusual foam or residue around the top. Sometimes it has a blue color, but if it is a dark drink

you won't be able to see it. Use your *taste buds* and remember this Safety Chick mantra: WHEN IN DOUBT, POUR IT OUT.

Too Close for Comfort

TIP #2 "HOW 'BOUT YOU COME BACK TO MY PLACE AND CHILL?"

- The easiest way to get out of an uncomfortable sexual setting is to not be there in the first place.

Acquaintance rape is a misunderstood form of criminal violence. There is a common misconception that acquaintance rape is not as serious, not as criminal, and not as traumatic to the victim as stranger rape. Some people think it isn't "real rape." These are mistaken beliefs. Rape is a felony crime, regardless of the offender's relationship to the victim. Acquaintance rape is just as serious and just as devastating to the victim as stranger rape.

If you are a victim of acquaintance rape, get the help and support you need to cope with the effects of the assault and heal from the trauma you have suffered.

One of the most important ways to avoid becoming a victim of rape is to avoid compromising situations. Be very careful if you have been drinking or using drugs. Your judgment will be clouded, and you could find yourself in a very dangerous setting. If you do find yourself in an uncomfortable situation, follow these guidelines from the Rape Treatment Center of Santa Monica—UCLA Medical Center & Orthopaedic Hospital.

Know your sexual intentions and limits and communicate them clearly:
You have the right to say "no" to any unwanted sexual contact. If you say "no," say it like you mean it. Back up your words with your body language. If you are uncertain about what you want, ask your partner to respect your feelings. Don't give mixed messages.

Don't assume your partner can read your mind:
Don't assume that your partner will get the message without having to say what you are feeling. Tell the person you are with how far you are willing to go, what you want and don't want to do, and when you want to stop.

Remember that some people think that drinking heavily, wearing "sexy" clothes, or agreeing to be alone with them indicates a willingness to have sex:
Be especially careful to communicate your limits and intentions clearly in such situations.

Trust your "gut" feelings:
If you start to feel uncomfortable or unsafe in a situation, listen to your feelings and act on them. Get yourself out of the situation as soon as possible.

Don't be afraid to ask for help or make a scene if you feel threatened:
If you are getting pressured or forced into sexual activity against your will, let the other person know how you feel and get out of the situation, even if it's awkward and even if you embarrass the other person or hurt his feelings.

Be especially careful in situations involving the use of drugs or alcohol:
Drugs and alcohol can make you less aware of danger signs and less able to communicate clearly. Be especially aware when you are in a new situation or with people that you don't know well. You need to be able to make good decisions to protect yourself from sexual assault.

Go to parties or clubs with friends you can trust and agree to look out for one another:
At parties where there is drinking or drugs, appoint a designated sober person, one friend who won't drink and who will look out for the others in the group by regularly checking on them. Leave parties with people you know. Don't leave alone or with someone you don't know very well.[3]

Buddy Up

TIP #3 SOBER SISTERS

- Always have a designated sober person when you go to parties, nightclubs, or any night on the town.

Always try to plan with a friend or two or a group for a party or other social event where there will be crowds and probably drinking and/or drugs. On the night of the event, have a "team meeting" before you leave. Get ready to have fun, but always have a sober buddy—someone who is designated to check up on you, and who you check in with throughout the night. A friend is not a policeman, but someone who is looking out for your best interest. Also plan to check in with each other every half hour or so; at the end of the night, arrange a meeting place to convene before going home.

[3] Reprinted with permission from the Rape Treatment Center of Santa Monica—UCLA Medical Center & Orthopaedic Hospital.

A Friend Doesn't Let Her Friend Go Home with the Stranger at the Bar

I have talked about this in other places in the book, but this truth bears repeating: No matter how cute and sexy he is, you just can't trust a stranger. If you want to encourage your friend's new interest, tell her to get the guy's phone number and call him the next day; NEVER let her go home with someone she just met, or even someone she knows but not well. Protect your sisters!

A Friend Gets Immediate Medical Attention If a Friend Appears Extremely Intoxicated

If your friend appears very intoxicated after only a few drinks, if she passes out or seems to have trouble breathing, or if she's not behaving like her normal self, get medical attention AT ONCE.

A Friend Warns Her Friends about High-Risk Situations

If you have heard that a club, frat house, or other party place has been known to put drugs into drinks, tell all of your friends and absolutely avoid that location. There are always other choices. If you end up in a place you think is safe but then see or hear that someone is dosing a drink or punch bowl, react! If there is security or other adult presence nearby, intervene and confront the person. Warn potential victims, discard the drinks, and get help. If your intuition tells you that the setting is dangerous, grab your friends, get out, and dial 911.

A Friend Trusts Her Friends' Intuition as Well as Her Own

As I have stated over and over throughout this book, intuition is the key to avoiding danger. The more intuition, the better; if your friend raises concerns, listen to her. Make safety decisions together.

What to Do If You've Been Drugged

If you suspect that you've been drugged, pay close attention to your body for a while; you might not feel anything for fifteen minutes or up to half an hour. Get medical help immediately if you start to feel funny. Pay attention if you feel unexpected sensations. The first noticeable signs of an uninvited drug in your system are often dizziness, drowsiness, confusion, impaired motor skills, and/or disorientation. If you feel like this and you've only had one cocktail (or maybe two if you are more experienced with alcohol), take action. The first thing to do is tell a friend. Have this person help you outside to a safe place and stay with you at all times. If you start feeling extremely ill, get to a hospital or call 911 for help. According to the Rape Treatment Center in Santa Monica, California, these drugs metabolize very quickly in your body. The sooner you get medical attention, the better chance you have of finding evidence of what you were drugged with. Request a urine test and set it aside for the police. If you have been drugged with Rohypnol, there is a reversing agent called Romazicon that can be administered by a doctor but it only works in cases of severe overdose.

What to Do If You Have Been Raped

If you have been raped or are the victim of any sexual assault, as soon as you can, get to a safe place and call the police. Call a trusted friend and have her stay with you and help you through this devastating and horrific time. Be sure to preserve all physical evidence of the assault—though you may feel a strong aversion, it is very important that you do not take a shower, do not change your clothes, do not wash your hands, or brush your teeth. If you suspect you were drugged, find the glass or bottle you were drinking from (but only if it is safe to do so). Every speck of evidence should be collected at the hospital by law enforcement professionals. Write down as much as you can remember of the incident and a description of the rapist. Make sure you do it right after the event, so little details are still fresh in your mind. The more evidence you have, the easier to convict the scumbag who did this to you.

You will find that the traumatic effects of a sexual assault will continue, often lingering in painful and confusing ways. Be sure to get emotional support from experts as well as friends and family—there are wonderful rape crisis centers all over the country that can assist you in getting the help that you need (see Resources, page 194).

FACT: Sexual intercourse with someone who is mentally or physically incapable of giving consent can be considered rape or sexual assault.

Safety Chick Checklist:
What to Do If You or a Friend Has Been Drugged

⊠ **SAVE ANY EVIDENCE |** Remember what beverage you were drinking and if you can, collect the glass, bottle, or anything that might contain evidence.

⊠ **GET TO A HOSPITAL EMERGENCY ROOM |** Tell the nurses that you think you have been drugged. Have them take a blood and urine sample and store it to be tested by police.

⊠ **CALL 911 |** Report drugging and possible rape to the police immediately. Have them meet you at the emergency room.

⊠ **TRY TO REMEMBER |** As soon as you can concentrate, write down names, descriptions of everyone that you interacted with, and any other details you can think of for possible witnesses or the drugger himself.

⊠ **GET ONGOING SUPPORT |** If you have been raped, contact a rape crisis center for help.

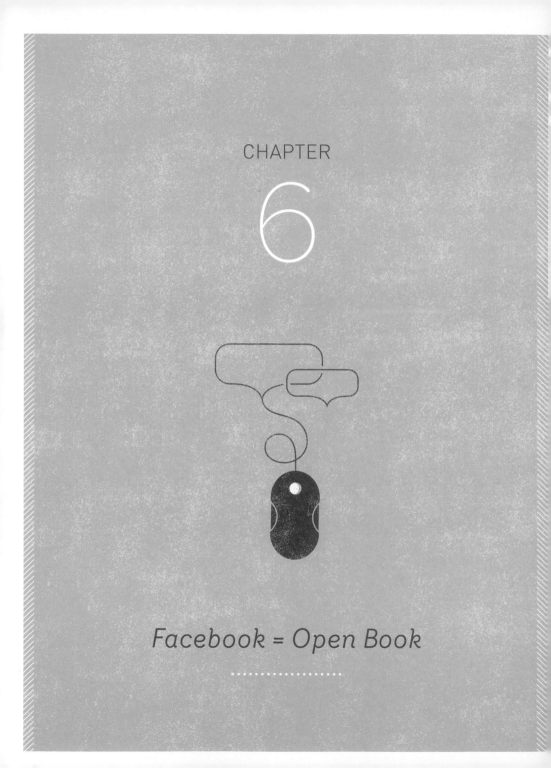

CHAPTER

6

Facebook = Open Book

Megan Meier was a beautiful Missouri teenager who met a boy on MySpace. He started writing her comments, saying how beautiful she was; how gorgeous her eyes were; that he was mesmerized by her beauty; and before long, that she was the only girl for him. She really grew to like him and was excited about the possibility of a budding romance. He said he had recently moved from Florida, was home-schooled, and knew a lot of the kids she went to high school with in O'Fallon, Missouri. The online flirting went on for few weeks. Then one day she came home to find a message on her MySpace that basically said he was no longer interested, that he had heard that she was not very nice to her friends. The next day, Megan's "cyber crush" cruelly wrote, "Everybody in O'Fallon knows how you are. You are a bad person and everybody hates you. Have a shitty rest of your life. The world would be a better place without you." What this guy did not realize is that Megan suffered from depression and low self-esteem. What this guy did not realize is that his mean and tormenting game would cause this beautiful, sweet, young teenager to lock herself in her bedroom, tie a rope around her neck, and hang herself from her closet door.

The most disturbing part of this story is the fact that the boy that Megan was communicating with on MySpace was not a boy at all. In fact, it was a group of people—unbelievably, led by the parents of one of her classmates, a former friend. They created a fake MySpace page to embarrass Megan, because they felt she was spreading rumors about them. They wanted to torment and humiliate her. Because of this horrific incident, the Megan Meier Cyberbullying Prevention Act HR 1966 was created. This act imposes criminal penalties on anyone who transmits in interstate or foreign commerce a communication intended to coerce, intimidate, harass, or cause emotional distress to another person using electronic means to support severe, repeated, and hostile behavior. The bill has not passed, but it certainly has created a lot of dialogue and attention in both media and political circles, bringing attention to this growing and troubling behavior.

The reason I am telling you this tragic story is to underscore that socializing on the Internet MUST be done responsibly. It's so casual, so available, so easy, and so everywhere. BUT its impact and outreach is vast, infinite. You need to think of socializing on the Internet like fishing in a big ocean. Until you reel in your rod and see for yourself, you have no idea what or who is on the end of the line. Could be a cute little red snapper, or it could be a big, mean, ugly shark. I will talk about social media more later in the chapter. Let's start now with the basics: securing your computer.

Internet Safety Basic Operations

The key to using the Internet is to try to maintain control of your personal information as well as maintaining who has access to that information. Tom Quilty of BD Consulting and Investigations Inc. is a risk management consultant (and an awesome Safety Dude) who has years of experience helping large corporations and global companies protect themselves from external IT security risks. He is a computer safety expert who spent eight of his twenty-five law enforcement years with the FBI REACT High Technology Crimes Task Force. He gave me some great, easy tips on securing your computer from the inside out.

The easiest way to start is by securing the device, computer, iPad, cell phone, etc., with a good password (minimum of eight, but preferably more, characters with at least one capital letter, number, and special character such as #, ~, #, !, etc.) and not using the Administrator account for normal activities. After securing your device with a strong password, go to the control panel to check on your "Internet Options." You're most likely familiar with it; otherwise, ask your favorite IT guru. If you're not using Internet Explorer, look for the preferences or Security Settings box for your Internet browser and go from there. The security menu will show the features that allow you to customize your settings and avoid breaches to your security.

Cookies: No, Not Chocolate Chip

Well known and loved as an old-fashioned tasty treat, in computer terms, cookies can be trouble. Picture a server putting a cookie jar (a file that contains information such as a unique ID and administrative information to make it easier for the Web site to assist you in connecting to their site) on your hard drive when you log onto their site. The Web server is then able to store what is technically called a "cookie" (personal information of every move you make on its site sent from your ISP—Internet Service Provider, such as Verizon, AT&T, Earthlink, or Comcast—to your hard drive) in the jar. Some sites can access the information any time they want. For true e-commerce business sites, this helps them in understanding and assisting their customer needs. But for businesses whose sole operation is to gather private information to sell to the highest bidder, your cookies can be a dangerous tool—and not for increasing your hip size. For this reason, be sure to "Clear Cookies" on a regular basis.

Where There's Smoke, There SHOULD Be Fire

Firewalls are software programs or network appliances that block intruders from penetrating your internal network. This is a fabulous and easy way to protect yourself from hackers or other deviant Internet users. Here are a few of the top-rated software programs: ZoneAlarm Extreme Security by Check Point Software Technologies, OutPost by Agnitum, and Norman Personal Firewall by Norman. Like any software security program, you have to know and understand the settings and then select those that best meet your needs. Any computer store can tell you more about the products and help you decide which one is best for you. They are relatively easy to install and are a must for Internet users.

A Word about Passwords

Whenever you are online, you have to deal with passwords. Everything from banking to shopping to socializing and sharing photos requires you to create a password. If someone gets a hold of your password, there is danger of them going onto Facebook, MySpace, or Twitter and using your account to post something embarrassing about you—or worse, stealing your identity for theft or fraud. As stated earlier, the best practice is to combine numbers and letters—a combo of capital and lower case—along with special characters and change them often. When choosing a password, don't use your friend's first or last name, pet's name, birth date, or other commonly known information. Consider a pass phrase such as: 1-H8t-BroOil#. Last but not least: DO NOT share your password with your BFF, boyfriend, roommate, sister, classmate, or anyone. That is not a smart personal-safety choice.

There is a cool product called ID Vault that you can attach to your computer—it looks like a little padlock and it plugs into a port. It encrypts your passwords, usernames, and credit card information securely on your PC. The ID Vault also logs you in without typing and creates a secure end-to-end connection between your PC and online accounts . . . it even comes in great colors, like bubblegum pink!

Social Media Savvy and Etiquette

Social media is one of the newest and greatest ways to stay in touch with friends and stay in tune with what is going on in the world, and it gives you limitless opportunities. MySpace, Facebook, Twitter, and Craigslist are all sites that were created in the last decade. These companies and networks allow you to easily do things that were never even possible before. Unfortunately, the real world has not caught up to the cyberworld just yet, which leaves the Internet much like the Wild West—untamed and very dangerous if you are not careful.

The most important thing to remember about using any type of social media is that anything you write, photograph, record, and send is out there forever. Even if you hit the Delete button, it never goes away. Someone will always be able to dig it up in cyberspace. But as long as you function in the social media world as you would in the real world, you shouldn't have any problems.

Facebook, Twitter, YouTube—YouNameIt!

Facebook, Twitter, and YouTube are currently three of the most widely used social media Web sites, and so this chapter starts with those. By the time this book hits the shelves, there will be dozens more. Here is the bottom line: The key to making these pages fun and safe for you and your friends lies in the security and privacy settings within the sites, along with good common sense. Every social site out there is or will be a bit different. The idea is to understand which settings you need to be concerned with within these electronic media and how to create a barrier between you and cyberspace, while still being available to your friends as well as educated exploration.

My friend Mary Kay Hoal is the founder of www.yoursphere.com, a social media Web site developed for children. Mary Kay and her team outline on her site that they "work very hard to make sure those using the site are who they say they are. They look at substantial amounts of data to verify identity and require parental consent to open an account. They also run all parents' names against a comprehensive identity verification and sex offender database. If the name is in the sex offender database, or the identity can't be verified, the account is blocked and the individual cannot enter the site."

Her philosophy is that by removing the anonymity that is traditionally found online, they can hold all members accountable for their behavior. This is dramatically different from how most social media sites work, where if someone is banned, they can merely sign in with a different account using an alias. I hope one day all social media sites will follow Mary Kay's lead and take this type of responsible approach.

I asked Mary Kay about the current security settings for Facebook, and how people could truly protect their privacy with all the different tabs and setting choices. She referred me to a great Web site called www.ReclaimPrivacy.org, founded by Randall Deich, a professional developer and educator. He and his team have created a useful privacy tool made specifically for Facebook Privacy Settings. Their mission is to "promote privacy awareness on Facebook and elsewhere," and the site provides a free tool for scanning all of your Facebook privacy settings. Not only does it show you the vulnerabilities in your privacy settings, it also directs you to the exact page where you can fix them. While this is an excellent way to protect yourself, I still recommend that you READ the Terms of Service (TOS) for each site. Understand what information they may be collecting and sharing with vendors or other sites.

Facebook

Facebook Savvy
As stated above, Privacy and Security settings are constantly being updated by most social media sites, so the best thing to do is be diligent about reviewing every tab or link that deals with your account, page, and membership on a regular basis. This might take a bit of time, but it is worth it.

Facebook Etiquette
Socializing online safely not only requires privacy settings, but basic common sense and everyday considerateness as well. Screen names, profile pictures, etc. can all lead to negative or dangerous outcomes if you don't follow basic etiquette.

And never write a mean or rude or threatening comment on someone's photo or post; this is not only hurtful, it may be punishable by law.

Facebook profile pictures—Trust me, you can have a cute profile picture and still have clothes on! I cannot tell you the number of pictures I have seen that would make you blush. Bottom line: If you wouldn't want your grandma, teacher, coach, parents, or boss to see it, don't put it on the Internet. First impressions say a lot. Make your photo represent who you are on the inside and out.

Facebook relationship status—I don't know about you, but I would be devastated if my boyfriend broke up with me by changing the status on his Facebook page from "in a relationship" to "single." Not only is this a cruel and cowardly thing to do, but if the person you're breaking up with is unstable, it could be a catalyst for violent behavior. Don't communicate personal or hurtful information by changing your status—talk to the person first.

Twitter

Twitter Savvy

Using Twitter allows you to get short messages out instantly, keeps you current on your favorite topic, and allows you to interact with virtually thousands of people all at one time—all of which is exactly why you must follow certain safety guidelines when tweeting.

There are many common mistakes that people make on Twitter. Getting caught up in the frenzy of tweeting your every move can be dangerous. It can make you a target for criminals. One man told every detail of his family's vacation—when they were leaving, where they were going, when they were returning, etc. The family arrived home to find their house totally empty. A burglar had known where they lived and calmly went in and cleaned out their house. All because of a few tweets! So here are a few things to remember:

Protect your tweets—Just like all social networking pages, be sure to set the security settings. Go to the security page and click the Protect My Tweets box.

Beware the TinyUrl—These little guys are the product of a free Internet service that converts long, unwieldy URL's into short tidy ones for e-mail links. Before you click, make sure you know the source of a URL within a tweet. Clicking on a short URL can lead to malware, or phishing—which can infect your computer with a virus or attempt to steal your personal information from Web sites.

Direct Message Warning—Be careful of unsolicited DM's. These can also be phishing attacks (see above) to lure unsuspecting users to a fake login page, where they ask for your password and User ID to hack into your account.

Twitter Etiquette

Remember: Tweeting is the same as speaking out loud for the whole world to hear!

Live in the past—It's okay to talk about a trip you went on, a place you visited . . . but do it AFTER you get home, not before or while you are there.

TMI—Do not discuss personal things or use full names. Think of using Twitter as giant a billboard on an extremely busy highway—don't write anything you wouldn't feel comfortable with posted on that billboard.

No Impostors—Pretending to be someone else on Twitter can be funny, but one day might also be considered a crime. Some people use other people's identities to harass them or gain personal information from others. If you think someone is using your identity on Twitter, send the Web administrator an e-mail at impersonation@twitter.com and report it immediately.

YouTube

Making videos with your friends and then being able to post them online—how's that for simply amazing technology! I have seen so many funny and creative things. It is also amazing how much crap is out there—stuff that I am sure many people wish they hadn't posted but thought it was a good idea at the time. Here are some basic security steps to follow when making, recording, or posting videos online.

YouTube Savvy

Be aware of what's in back—The background of your video can give away a lot of personal information. Be aware of family photos or signs that reveal names or contact information. If you are outside, stay away from showing where you live; the front of your sorority house or dorm, even your car's license plate can give strangers too much info.

Respect the copyright—Don't use or post anything that has a copyright without permission. Do you remember Napster—the music site that got shut down with its founder in major hot water with the law after allowing people to download copyrighted material free on his site? The Internet is no different than the real world—using copyrighted material is against the law.

Watch where that cell phone is pointing—"Upskirting" is a disgusting crime that was quite popular a few years ago—a guy goes into a department store, hides under a clothing rack, and shoots videos with his camera up women's skirts on his cell phone, then posts it on the Internet for others to watch. Be aware of who is around you and where they are pointing their cell. You could become a victim of a crime without even knowing it—until it appears on YouTube.

YouTube Etiquette

As with all social media, YouTube etiquette is about being a responsible and good citizen. Making videos that make fun of or truly hurt another person is not where it's at.

Actions speak even louder than words—Be very careful about what you say or do in a video. Unlike an e-mail or post, it's pretty hard to dispute the face, body, and voice of someone ranting and raving on a video. In real-life terms, it's called slander, libel, or defamation—all prosecutable by law.

The camera doesn't lie—Please remember that anything you do on camera that is posted on the Internet can be used to incriminate you. Drinking under age, vandalizing something, bullying, or fighting can get you a visit from the police.

What do Paris Hilton, Pamela Anderson, and Kim Kardashian all have in common?—They all made a video that they wish they hadn't. I guarantee you none of these women thought their private sex tapes would be broadcast in front of god and everyone years later! Think BEFORE you strip . . . video lasts forever and ever and they always seem to pop up when you least expect them to.

Sexting Is Stupid

"Sexting" is a super-post-modern term for the act of sending sexually explicit messages or photos electronically, primarily through cell phones. As I write, the phenomenon is also considered a crime, and legislative response across states and around the world is teeming. Sending nude pictures of yourself or others can be considered child pornography if the subject of the photo is under the age of eighteen. The act of sexting can have a whole lot more than legal ramifications. These texts can ruin reputations and cause extreme humiliation if they fall into the wrong hands. Whether you are over eighteen or not, here are some things to consider before you snap that pic. (For more information, visit sextingisstupid.org.)

Whose Idea Was This, Anyway?

Taking a nude photo of yourself might not really be your idea. If you are feeling pressure from a boyfriend or others and really don't want to be doing it, then don't!

The Ex Factor

Taking nude pictures for your boyfriend's eyes only isn't always the case. A lot of guys can't resist sharing their good fortune (your hot body) with their friends. What if you break up with your boyfriend and he is not happy about it? Your privates could end up all over the school and Internet for revenge.

Fast Forward

If you receive a nude photo of someone, delete it. Do not forward it to ANYONE. It can be considered trafficking of child pornography if the person in the photo is under eighteen, and you can be prosecuted. More importantly, how do you know what was going on when the photo was taken? What if the person was being forced against her will, or was drunk and didn't fully understand what was going on? How would you feel if it was you? Remember: Do not forward— delete instead.

Cyberbullying and Cyberstabbing

By now, many people have heard of "cyberbullying," the word for when a person is tormented, threatened, or harassed by another person by use of the Internet, digital technologies, or mobile phones. Cyberbullying is most common among elementary or high school kids. For the Safety Chick handbook, I want to define a specific subset of cyberbullying that has become lamentably common among college women. I call it "cyberstabbing." This is the same thing as backstabbing or gossiping, but it happens online. Remember when we talked about mean girls in the sisterhood chapter (page 54)? This goes back to that same principle. Talking about someone on a friend's page or posting mean comments about her might be considered defamation of character and could possibly be punishable by law. So it is very important NOT to get caught up in this kind of behavior. Following are examples of some situations that could get you into trouble or involved in something you don't want to be a part of.

Gossip Girl

Would you ever walk into your English class and announce that the guy sitting next to you made out with your roommate last night? Especially if her boyfriend was in the same class, too? Posting gossip and hearsay online is essentially the same idea, except to a larger audience. Forwarding negative messages or posts even if you didn't write them still makes you an accomplice.

You Are Who You Associate With

Be very careful about joining groups on Facebook and other Web sites. If a group or club participates in hateful or discriminating speech or threatening or illegal behavior, and you are a member—you are guilty as well. Do your research before you join.

Stop It in Its Tracks

You know when words cross the line. Practice zero tolerance. Do not participate, and report any harassment, gossip, or abuse to the proper channels.

What to Do If You Are a Victim

Words are very powerful and can be extremely hurtful or abusive. Hearing someone say negative things about you, whether in person or through the grapevine, is tough. Having them posted on the Internet by someone you know (or not) can be even worse. Here are some tips to help you if you are being cyberstabbed online.

Don't Bite

If someone is sending you mean e-mails, texts, or other messages, don't respond. I know it can be frustrating not to fire back, but it only makes matters worse. The harasser wants to get a reaction out of you, which is usually her goal in the first place. A lot of times the harasser will get bored or frustrated and simply go away.

Do NOT Hit Delete

If you are being threatened or harassed online, save all the messages, posts, comments, photos, etc. You need evidence to show to the authorities. You also might need them to back up requests for blocking and reporting the online abuse to the various service providers.

Speak UP

Being a victim of cyberstabbing or any kind of harassment can be emotional and embarrassing. Don't let the cybercowards get you down! Take charge and stand your ground. Immediately report the incident to the appropriate social media company and block the harasser or group. Talk to someone about it—your parents, an administrator, or other authority figure that you trust.

Know Your Rights
Being threatened or taunted or harassed by someone, whether it's online or in person, is a crime. Check with local authorities to find out what your rights are and if you are a victim of a crime.

Internet Dating Safety

It seems sort of unlikely to me that you will be interested in an online dating service with all of the guys roaming around your college campus—and with everything else you've got to do! But it is certainly a means for meeting people and for making connections that may not be happening otherwise, and if handled—note the emphasis here—*very* carefully, it can be a valid and safe resource for young women. If you decide to check out online dating, there are a few things that you need to know. First of all, you need to be over eighteen. Second, while first dates of any kind can be a bit tricky, meeting someone over the Internet requires some serious precautions. Be sure to use a reputable dating service, one that uses "anonymizers" and re-mailers, software programs that will hide your real e-mail address.

Safety Guidelines for Meeting Your Cybermatch in Person

When meeting any stranger for the first time, always do so in a public place—even if he is a friend of a friend of yours. Start with a "meet and greet" during the day for coffee or a soda. Short and sweet, so you can size him up and make sure he is who he says he is. Stick to the following guidelines.

Bring a Friend
It's always a good idea to bring someone along the first time you meet your cyberdate in person. Meet him at a public location. Do NOT let him come to your house and pick you up. You don't want him knowing where you live until you actually *know* he's not an axe murderer!

No TMI
Do not give out too much personal information about yourself. Give it a few dates before you tell him where you want to get married and how many kids you want. Seriously, get to know the guy better before you share personal details about your life.

Tell a Friend

If your friend can't come along, be sure to tell her or a parent as much information about your date as you can: where you are meeting him, what time, and any description or details you have about him. Tell her you will check in when you arrive at the location and when you leave. Don't forget to do it—you wouldn't want her calling 911 by mistake!

Watch for Tan Lines

If you see a tan line around his left ring finger, that's a pretty good indication the guy might be married. Be sure to ask all the necessary questions before you unknowingly get into a relationship with a married man.

Trust Your Instincts

Always trust your intuitive body signals (see Chapter 1). Use that gut instinct to tell if something is amiss. If you show up and the guy is a complete creep, leave immediately and notify the dating service. You can protect other vulnerable women from a stressful time or real trouble.

I have covered A LOT of material in this chapter. And, as I have said before, by the time this book hits the shelves, some of the technology will inevitably have changed. The most important thing to remember about ANY cyber or digital media is: Once it is out there, it is out there FOREVER. No Delete button in the world can erase a photo, text, e-mail, or any other electronic missive once it is out in cyberspace. So always act wisely.

Safety Chick Checklist:
Staying Safe on the Internet

✖ **FIGHT WITH FIRE** | Secure your computer with firewalls and security settings.

✖ **KEEP IT IMPERSONAL** | Do not share personal information with strangers over the Internet.

✖ **BE SOCIALLY SMART** | Make sure all your social media pages are secure and private.

✖ **BE THE FIRST ON YOUR BLOCK** | Immediately block and report any abusers.

✖ **THINK BEFORE YOU HIT SEND** | Remember, what goes out in cyberspace is there FOREVER.

CHAPTER

7

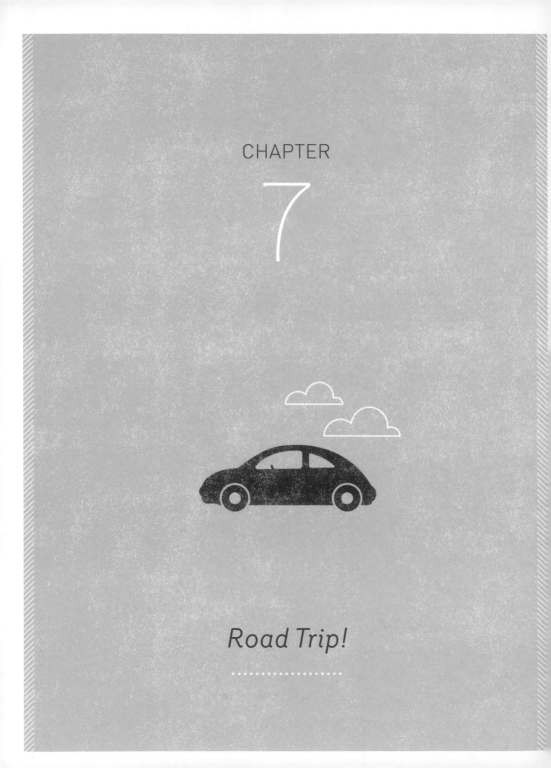

Road Trip!

One weekend during my college days, my sorority decided to have a big party at a hotel in Palm Springs. The drive was about two and a half hours from the UCLA campus. One of my friends volunteered to drive four of us down. We were about forty-five minutes away, in the middle of the desert, when her car started making a weird noise. The next thing we knew, the car sputtered to a stop on the side of the freeway. Luckily, we were about a quarter mile from an exit with a gas station. As it turned out, there was some sort of hose broken on the car and the gas station mechanics didn't have the part and they couldn't get it until the next day. We were stranded in a small town in the middle of nowhere, with a flea-bag motel as our only shelter for the night. Luckily, we did not encounter any trouble as we huddled together walking down the freeway ramp. We ended up missing the party, but were very happy to arrive in one piece. The lesson learned: before you go on a road trip, get your car checked out by a mechanic to make sure everything is in working order.

One of the most storied annals of great college memories is road trips with friends, whether driving to a rival college for a football game or going away for Spring Break or traveling abroad for a semester. However, again—and always remembering that smart doesn't mean paranoid—making a small investment in time to learn about travel safety can be the difference between life and death. We need look no further back than to the tragic story of Natalee Holloway, the high school senior who disappeared on a graduation trip to Aruba in 2005. She left a bar with some local guys and was never seen alive again. No one was ever prosecuted in the case, and her family and friends were left devastated. College trips can be wonderful adventures, but there are many dangers that come with being unprepared.

If you are a scuba diver, you know the expression "Plan your dive, dive your plan." What that means is know where you are going and what you need to do. DO NOT arrive in a city without hotel reservations. DO check the weather in advance (what a great modern convenience—you sure don't want to be driving around an unfamiliar town in a blizzard). DO get a map of the city you will be traveling in before you leave, so you can become familiar with the area. Search the Internet and call a travel agency or a tourism board to get all the information you need for the places you will be visiting.

The tips in the following pages will help you earn your scouting merit badges for travel.

How to Pack: The Basics

- If you need a Smarte Carte to carry your bags, you packed too much.

Unless you are a "celebutante" traveling with your own personal staff, packing for a trip takes some thought and organization so that you will have what you need, but can still carry all of your things by yourself. Whether you are headed to the Big Apple or backpacking around Europe, your knapsack or suitcase can get very heavy after a few days of schlepping it around. Traveling light also means less stuff to worry about getting ripped off.

What to Pack

Make sure that you have these essential items in your bag before you leave:

- **Flashlight**—Always tuck a flashlight in your suitcase, and make sure it has fresh batteries. You never know when the power might go out in your hotel or you will need to read a road map.
- **Medication**—Remember to bring any medication you are currently taking. Keep it with you, not in your suitcase. You do not want to become separated from vital medication, especially if you can become incapacitated or ill without it.
- **Boo-boo strips**—Bring a first-aid kit (Band-aids, aspirin, antibiotic ointment, etc.)—you don't want to have to make a drugstore run in the middle of the night in a strange city.
- **Alarm clock**—Carry a battery-operated alarm clock. You can't always trust a wake-up call from the front desk, and if the power goes off in the hotel, you'll want to know how long until daylight.

- **Calling card**—If you know you will be traveling in a region where there is no cell service, or you don't have a cell phone, purchase a prepaid calling card ahead of time and always carry it with you. Somehow, you never seem to have change when you need it.

- **Emergency contact list**—Don't forget a list of emergency contacts. Keep the list, along with all your important business and personal documents, in the hotel safe. In case anything should to happen to you, hotel personnel or the police will be able contact your family or your doctor.

- **Passport**—Be sure to keep your passport up to date, and have a photocopy of your passport and an extra passport picture (you know, the one that looks like a mug shot). If you lose your passport, these can help expedite the replacement process.

What Not to Pack

- **Valuables**—If you bring your iTouch, iPhone, iWHATEVER—watch them like a hawk. Traveling with valuables is like taking a spin on the roulette wheel. I recommend leaving the nice stuff at home.

  If you must take valuables, carry them on your person—do not pack them in your suitcase. You never know, your luggage could be lost or stolen. Once you are in your hotel, lock any valuables in the hotel safe. When you are traveling, you want to blend in, not stick out. Keep your bling to a minimum; leave the shiny stuff at home. You don't want to be a beacon for thugs on the street.

- **The Slouchy Hobo Bag**—You'll need to carry a sensible purse, something that closes with a secure clasp and can be worn diagonally across your shoulder so that the purse is in front of your body. The cute backpack thing is definitely a no-no when traveling. Backpacks are a pickpocket's dream. Great travel purses are the ones that lie flat on your chest and have a wide strap that crosses over your shoulder and around your back. These are tough for robbers to rip or cut off your body. Remember, the more difficult you make it for the criminals, the more likely they will leave you alone. These types of bags and purses are easy to find—readily available at handbag shops, department stores, travel stores, and tons of places online.

Taxis, Trains, and Automobiles: How to Get from Point A to Point B

If you are flying into a city late at night, you should arrange for a licensed car service to pick you up at your arrival terminal. If you don't already have the name of a car service in your destination city, call the hotel where you will be staying and ask for a recommendation. That way, you know that your transportation has been arranged and the company is legitimate. It also saves the time and hassle of getting a cab or other form of transportation at a crowded terminal. Some hotels have their own buses or mini-vans. Find out ahead of time where to meet your shuttle and how often it runs. By arranging for a driver to pick you up in advance, you have the comfort and safety of knowing that someone will be waiting for you.

"TAXI!"

Taxicabs are one of the easiest and safest ways to get around in a big city. Aside from their sometimes scary driving skills, cabbies can be quite entertaining and informative.

Taxi Savvy

If you are in an airport, ask at the information desk or follow signs to the taxi stands. Large cities regulate the number of taxis on the street. If you don't find one to flag, look for taxi stands in high-traffic areas, or look for a hotel with one. In smaller cities, you will probably have to find a phonebook and call for a cab.

Before you enter a cab, be sure to ask the driver what the current metered rate is for taxis, so you have a rough idea of what your fare will be (don't forget to use your economic intuition to sense if the meter is running too fast and you are getting ripped off). Like anything else, a few bad apples—in this case, fraudulent cab drivers—can spoil the batch. Make sure you are in a legitimate taxi by checking as soon as you enter for the driver's registered cab company license, called a "medallion." This looks like a license or credential with the company name, state or city seal, and photo and name of the driver. It is usually displayed on the dashboard or on one of the visors.

Let's Make a Deal

In some foreign countries, there are NO regulations. Anyone who owns a car can be a taxi driver—this makes it a dog-eat-dog business, which can be quite dangerous for visitors. Foreign taxi drivers love tourists because they consider them easy money. All fares are negotiable, so ask your driver what the fare will be and come to an agreement BEFORE you step in the cab. Again, it's also a good idea to have the hotel arrange a car service, so you know it is a reputable company. Ask the concierge or desk clerk what the going fares are, so you can be a little more informed before the foreign cabbie takes you for a ride.

Safety Chick Checklist: Taxi Tips

⊠ **ALWAYS USE AN ESTABLISHED COMPANY**

⊠ **ASK WHAT THE RATE IS BEFORE YOU GET INTO THE CAB.**

⊠ **DO NOT SHARE A CAB WITH SOMEONE YOU DO NOT KNOW.**

⊠ **DO NOT SHARE PERSONAL INFORMATION** with the cab driver; keep the topic of conversation on the weather or local places of interest. (Use your intuition. If you're uncomfortable, or if something isn't right with the driver, get out of the cab.)

⊠ **ALWAYS MAKE A NOTE** of the cab number and driver's name and license number (words cannot describe the feeling of watching your wallet drive away into a sea of yellow taxis).

⊠ **MAKE SURE THAT THE METER READS $0** when you start your trip. If not, politely ask your driver to reset the meter.

⊠ **TELL THE DRIVER YOU WOULD LIKE TO TAKE THE MOST DIRECT ROUTE.** Take a map and plot your path so you know where the driver should be taking you.

⊠ **PUT A BUSINESS CARD OR MATCHBOOK OF YOUR HOTEL IN YOUR PURSE BEFORE YOU LEAVE** so you can be assured that you will return to the right place. (Do you know how many Hyatts there are in New York City?)

⊠ **DO NOT GET OUT OF A CAB IN A DARK, DESOLATE, OR POORLY LIT AREA.** Make sure the driver drops you off right in front of your destination.

Trains and Subways

When you are using the subway or metro train, try really hard not to look like a tourist. Standing in the middle of a subway station staring at a large map of the city makes you a beacon for cruising criminals. Plan your destinations before you leave your hotel. Have the concierge or front desk clerk help you out with directions and train schedules. If you have questions once you're in the station, ask the clerk selling the tickets or tokens. Once again, keep an eye on those personal belongings. Subways and train stations are usually very crowded—purses are stolen in the blink of an eye and the thief easily disappears into the crowd.

Go into the Light

Don't ever get into an empty subway car. Remember: Safety in numbers. If you find yourself in an empty car, simply exit at the next stop and switch to a crowded one. The best place to sit on a subway is in the front middle of the train. Look for the blue light on top of the car. This is usually where the conductor stands and regulates the comings and goings of the passengers. If any problems were to arise, he would be the first person to call security and take care of the matter.

Subway Car Etiquette

Riding on the subway is quite a unique experience. While it's fun to do a character study of the people who ride, it's best not to make eye contact. Pay attention to where you are so you don't miss your stop. In some countries, eye contact can mean a whole lot more to a man than, "My gosh, that's cheap cologne you're wearing." Watch yourself—many women have been groped on train and subway cars. Some men will take any opportunity to cop a feel. If this happens to you, make a loud objection, complete with hand gestures. In any language, the point gets across.

Rental Cars

I realize that at this point you might not be old enough to rent a car, but in a few years you will be, or you might be traveling with a friend who is old enough to rent, so pass these tips on to her.

Back Off, Bucko

Many criminals wait around car rental lobbies to eavesdrop on your personal information, such as credit card or driver's license numbers. Remember to be aware of people standing around you. Fill out your rental forms on your own—don't shout out your personal information to the agent. Hand him your credit card and driver's license and let him punch the information into the computer.

Night Moves

Don't ever rent a car at night. There usually are only one or two employees on staff, and getting to your car in a dark parking lot isn't very safe. It's also difficult to get your bearings when driving in an unfamiliar town in the dark. If you get in late, take a cab to your hotel and rent your car in the morning.

Baby, You Can Drive My Car

Have the rental car agent show you exactly where your car is. You don't want to be wandering around the parking lot, looking for your slot number. Once you have reached your car, get in, lock your doors, and take your time familiarizing yourself with all the knobs and switches. Do you know how to turn on the lights? How about the windshield wipers? (Recently I was caught by surprise when I was on vacation in Florida. It started raining REALLY hard and I couldn't find the windshield wipers—I almost took out a whole line of palm trees.)

Adjust your seat and all the mirrors before you put your car in drive. Check the gas tank—is it full? Which side of the car is the gas tank on? These are important details to note *before* you pull out of the parking lot. You don't want to be stranded on the side of the road—out of gas, in a strange city. Once you've picked a jamming radio station (not too loud—you want to be aware of your surroundings), you're ready to hit the road. Don't forget to have change for tolls you might encounter on the way.

Details, Details

Be sure to write down the make, model, color, and license plate number of your vehicle. It's usually on the key chain, but if you lose it or something happens to the car, you will need that information for the rental company. Don't advertise that you are a tourist. Leave all maps and brochures of tourist traps like the Wax Museum in the glove compartment, and lock your luggage and valuables in the trunk.

Hotel Safety

Staying at a hotel with a bunch of girlfriends is so much fun. Nothing better than cramming as many people as you can into one room to save on hotels bills! But with that fun, comes responsibility—not only for the room itself, but for each other. Follow these essential tips when checking into any hotel.

Arriving

First, if you have a car, pull right up to the front to check in. If there is a bellman on duty, he will help you with your bags. If the hotel does not have a bellman, pull up to the front to check in and leave your car there while you unload your bags (do not leave your keys in the car, and lock your doors). Go register, get your bags to your room, and then park your car. Park close to the front entrance and in a well-lit area. Again, be aware of your surroundings (your intuition should *really* be kicking in about now; see page 14). Is anyone lurking around the parking lot? If so, don't get out of your car. Once again, drive to the front of the hotel and get one of the employees to escort you to and from your car.

Hotel, Motel, Holiday Inn

While most college students are on budgets and staying at a cheap motel is tempting, a motel poses bigger safety issues than a larger hotel. Most motels are open and the door to your room is usually right next to cars parked in the lot. Never park in a space that has a number to match your room number; with that system, anyone can watch you leave your space and break into your room while you're away; or worse, wait for you to return. Explain to the desk manager that for safety reasons you wish to park in either an unmarked space or one with a different number.

Location, Location, Location

Another problem with motels is that they often don't employ the security measures of a conventional hotel. For example, most hotels have security guards on duty at all times; motels usually only have the front desk clerk. Any problems that arise would require a call to the local police—and who knows how long it would take for them to get there?

Additionally, most motels are only one or two stories, and most rooms have windows facing public areas. This can make it very easy for criminals to break into a room. If you must stay at a motel, try to stay on the upper floor, and close to the front office. Make sure there are outside lights right by your door and that your car is parked close by in a well-lit area. If you are in a hotel, request a room between the fourth and sixth floors, that does not have a connecting door. Why? A very interesting piece of safety trivia: many Fire Department ladders will not reach beyond the sixth floor. And four floors up is high enough to put you out of reach of most casual break-ins from the outside faces of the building. Make sure your room is by a heavily trafficked area such as an elevator or vending machine. It might be loud, but the more people milling about, the safer you are. Criminals like to strike in isolated areas.

Jeepers, Creepers, Make Sure to Use Your Peepers

Whether you're staying in a motel or a hotel, always look around before you enter your room. Make sure no one is following you. If you're concerned, immediately go back to the front desk or manager's office and get an employee to escort you to your room. (Remember: A savvy Safety Chick is never afraid to ask for help.) Do not leave your room before looking outside, either through the peephole or out the window. If someone is lurking around, call the front desk or wait for the stranger to leave.

Register Safely

When filling out the hotel registration card, put either J. Jones or Mr. and Mrs. Jones. Look, I'm as independent as the next gal, but let's face it—you don't want to advertise that you are a young woman (or group of young women) staying alone. It just isn't worth the risk. When the clerk is giving you your room key, ask him not to announce the number. Have him write it on a piece of paper and hand it to you. Instruct the front desk never to give out your name or room number. Ask the clerk to call you and tell you if someone inquires about you. Don't leave your credit card lying on the counter. Hand it directly to the front desk clerk, and make sure he hands you back the right credit card. (Many a con has been pulled at the front desks of hotels—the criminals either lurk behind you to copy down your credit card information or steal your purse or bags while you are busy registering.) Watch your back.

Find Your Room

Ask to be escorted to your room, either by a bellman or front desk clerk. Even if you are with a group of your girlfriends, have the bellman go with you in case there is a problem. As you walk to your room, note where the emergency exits are, as well as fire alarms and extinguishers. When you arrive at your room, ask the bellman or clerk to wait while you look around the room. Check that there is no one in the room—under the bed or in the closet or bathroom. Make sure that all the deadbolts, locks, windows, and telephone are functioning, and that the door securely closes. Once you have established that everything is in working order, tip the nice bellman and unpack your bags. Put all your valuables in the hotel safe and lock it. Put that safety flashlight and battery-operated alarm clock by the bed (see "What to Pack," page 102). Now, relax and get down to the pool!

Who's That Knockin' on My Door?

If someone knocks at your door, regardless of whether you are staying at a hotel or motel, look through the peephole and do not open the door if you do not recognize the face staring back at you. If you are not expecting room service or a visitor, ask who it is and what he wants. If he is someone claiming that he is from the hotel and needs to work on something, ask for his name and call the front desk first. If they are truly legitimate, he will not mind waiting. If it is a stranger, tell him you do not want to be disturbed and report him to the front desk.

Noise is a great crime deterrent. Put a lamp or chair in front of the door in your room and underneath the windows—use any objects that will make a racket if knocked over during an attempted break-in. —from SecurityWorld.com

Gimme a Sign

Once you have freshened up and are ready to go out and see the sights, make sure you take your room key, a matchbook or hotel business card with the hotel address and phone number on it, and any money or valuables that you did not lock in the hotel safe. When you leave your room, leave on the television and put a "do not disturb" sign on your door. If thieves think that someone is in the room, they are less likely to try to break in while you're gone.

Going Up?

As you make your way down to the lobby, when the elevator doors open, don't enter if there's just one other person inside. Remember: safety in numbers. If you feel uncomfortable or your intuition is telling you something is not right, wait for another car instead of taking your chances with a stranger in an elevator. If you find yourself in a potentially violent situation, press several buttons so the car will stop at each floor, allowing you to get out as soon as you can.

Safety R&R

If you decide to get some rest and relaxation by the pool, first put up your flag to signal the waitress that you would like to order a nice, cool beverage, then pull out your magazines. If you've brought the magazines from home, tear off the mailing label and rip it into tiny pieces so no one can get ahold of your dorm, apartment, or sorority address.

Most hotel personnel find it refreshing when people initiate their own personal safety. Do not be embarrassed or paranoid about following these safety tips. You will find that the hotel staff will be extremely accommodating and think of you as a savvy, empowered Safety Chick.

On the Road

As the story at the beginning of this chapter served to show, the key to staying safe on the road is to be prepared and make sure your car is in working order. Before you head out on a road trip adventure make sure you have taken the time to take care of business.

Get a Checkup

Have a certified mechanic give your car a once over. Have him check all the hoses, fluid levels, tire pressure, etc. Also, have him give you a little "Car Engine 101" to show you how and where to check the washer fluid, oil, water, air-conditioner fluid, tire pressure, etc. Every independent Safety Chick should know her way around a motor—even how to change a spare, although it is safer and a whole lot easier to call AAA or OnStar. You should definitely pony up for membership with one of these excellent road service emergency assistance companies if you're doing a road trip of any distance. They are one call away, with (usually) pretty fast response time, when you need a tow truck to change a tire when on the road. Always have an emergency road kit in your car as well, complete with jumper cables, flares, first aid kit, flashlight, rain poncho, blankets, and gloves.

The Paper Chase

Make sure your insurance, inspection, and registration are up to date. Have your insurance card, registration papers, and emergency numbers readily available in your glove compartment.

Get a Map

When you and your friends take a road trip, make sure you know the best roads to take. Do not take a shortcut if you are not absolutely positive where you are going. Also, think about the weather. Could there be snow over a mountain pass? Does it look like rain? Walking in a winter wonderland—NOT!!!

I did a segment on *The Montel Williams Show* a few years ago about staying safe when on the road. We were highlighting the tragic story of a family who was driving from San Francisco to Oregon and took a shortcut through the mountains. It began snowing really hard and the car became stuck in the snow. There was nothing around for miles.

The father decided to try to walk back to the main road for help. The mom and her two young daughters stayed in the car. He became lost and disoriented, and, tragically, died in the elements. The mother and her daughters were ultimately rescued, but devastated by the loss of a husband and father.

If your car breaks down in the snow, do not get out and attempt to find help. Use your cell phone or OnStar to call for help. Have your AAA card handy and the location of your vehicle. Look for landmarks or road markers to identify where you are. Do NOT keep the car running and the heater going. Instead, heat the car to a comfortable temperature, then turn off the car and stay warm with the blankets in your emergency car kit. You want to conserve gasoline.

Spring Break

If you ask most college students, spring break means surf, sand, and lots of bikinis and beach balls flying around. Dancing and partying on *MTV's Spring Break* completes the picture. The most common destinations are Florida, the Bahamas, or Mexico. But before you book your beach paradise, there are a few things that you need to be aware of to make sure that your good time is a safe time. As I mentioned earlier, Natalee Holloway's tragic story reminds all of us that a lot can happen on group trips. It is important not to take your safety for granted just because you are on an organized tour. It is still your responsibility to make smart personal-safety choices and look out for yourself and your friends.

Spring Break Basics

Follow these guidelines before you book your group spring break vacation:

Round Up a Posse

Pick a group of reliable friends to travel with. Make sure you are all compatible and have the same ideas in mind when it comes to the plans for the trip. Discuss the buddy system with everyone and the importance of safety in numbers.

Pick a Partner

Each day assign two friends to each other—the old-fashioned but effective buddy system. That way, one is always responsible for the other, making it easier to know where everyone is at all times and avoiding the confusion of who saw whom last.

Get Referrals

Ask other college friends or older peers about their Spring Break trips and get recommendations on where to go and what companies to use.

Choose a Reliable Company

There are several travel agencies and groups that organize Spring Break trips. Make sure that you pick one that is reputable. Spring Break Travel is one of the largest, and they have tons of package deals—you can even book an MTV package that gets you on the show! (See Resources, page 194.)

Get It in Writing

Before you pay any money, be sure to get all the travel details in writing. Read the fine print of any contract and get travel insurance. Also, pay with a credit card; that way, if there is any trouble with the company, you can cancel or dispute payment.

Once the plans have been made and the reservations are booked, be sure to do these three things to stay connected to home and in case of emergency:

1. Leave a copy of your daily itinerary with your parents, another family member, or a close friend. Check in with them on a daily basis so they know you are safe. Also, leave a copy of your passport with them in case yours gets lost and you need to get another.

2. Make sure your cell phone works where you are going. If it doesn't, buy a prepaid calling card or rent a cell phone. Skype, a free Internet-driven phone and video chat service, is also a wonderful way to stay in touch if you have access to a computer. All you have to do is download the software and you can talk for free. You'll also need a webcam if you want to use the video chat feature.

3. Bring your medical insurance card and any allergy or medical information you might need. If you take medication, bring enough for the time that you're gone—you don't want to run out and not be able to fill the prescription.

Spring Break South of the Border—I'm Gonna Sit Right Here and Have Another Beer In Mexico

In Mexico, the Bahamas, and many other countries, the drinking age is eighteen. So, for some of you, it will be the first time you can legally drink. Which means it might be the first time you have alcohol—which means you need to be really, really careful with your alcohol intake. The majority of accidents, injuries, and trouble on spring break happen because kids are intoxicated. (See Chapter 6 for more on the dangers of alcohol and drugs.) Here are a few special cautions and other advice regarding drinking and nonalcoholic concerns that go along with fun in the sun.

If Your Drink Has an Umbrella and Whipped Cream on Top, It Isn't Necessarily "Just" a Milkshake

Beware of those cute little froufrou drinks that taste like strawberry or coconut. Just because you can't taste the alcohol doesn't mean that there is no rum or vodka in it. These drinks are strong and dangerous. Know your limit, and only have one or two over a few hours. Drink plenty of bottled water to stay hydrated, as well.

Passing Out in the Sun Can Leave More than Bad Tan Lines

Don't let general giddiness, laziness, a wonderful sense of contentment, or a cold beer make you forget to wear lots and lots of sunscreen. A bad sunburn is painful at best, and at worst can equal sun poisoning. Symptoms of sun poisoning can include nausea, fever, headache, and dizziness and may also be accompanied by fluid loss and electrolyte imbalance, not a fun way to spend your vacation.

Don't Lose Your Balance

Many tragic accidents have happened when Spring Breakers—whether because of drinking or just crowding, horsing around, etc.—fall off balconies or roofs. Stay away from the edges of high places and for Pete's sake—stay off any hotel or building roofs!

Do Use Your Brain

Too much alcohol and dozens of crazy college kids can sometimes lead to bad decisions. Sexual assault or a bad sexual experience is all too common on spring break. The last thing you want to do is end up on a "Girls Gone Stupid" video and have to explain years later to your kids why you thought it was a good idea to flash your boobs for all the world to see.

Midnight Swim

Too much alcohol can impair your swimming ability and coordination. If you have been drinking, do not go for a swim at night and, even in the day, stay in the shallow water. There have been several drowning tragedies on spring break vacations.

It's a Long Trip Alone

Getting into trouble in a foreign country is extremely dangerous. American law does not apply and you could end up being locked up for a long, long time. Stay out of trouble and stay away from drunk, stupid, and belligerent college kids looking for trouble. You do not want to take a chance of being in the wrong place at the wrong time and ending up in a jail cell.

Be Active, But Smart

There are many fun and exciting activities to do while on Spring Break. If you want to do more than just hang by the pool or beach all day, use the hotel or travel group's recommendations for tour companies. For example, if you want to tour the island you are on, don't use just any tour guide, especially one who approaches you; make sure he is known by the hotel. Cons and thieves have a perfect scam pretending to be tour guides—once they have someone in a van or car, they can take her to a desolate area and rob her blind, or worse.

Spring Break is no different than any other time you travel. Remember to always have a buddy, watch out for each other, make smart personal-safety choices, and don't forget the sunscreen!

Wanna Get Away? Studying Abroad

There are many reasons to take a semester or a summer and travel overseas. Whether it's for personal growth, getting a new perspective on global affairs, or even to enhance your major or career path, Study Abroad programs are a fantastic way to see the world. If you are interested, the best thing to do is check out your school's Study Abroad office for more information. Most universities also have a travel or Study Abroad section with books on various programs and countries that have college programs. StudyAbroad.com is one of the largest online resources for Study Abroad programs; they can connect you with any Study Abroad organizations. Be sure to get references from your university and peers about the program you are selecting. To ensure your health and safety overseas, follow StudyAbroad.com's excellent tips and guidelines.

Bring the Records

It's a good idea to bring a copy of your medical and dental records with you. If you have any ongoing medical or dental problems, bring a letter from your doctor or dentist explaining how they are being treated. Don't forget the telephone and fax numbers of your doctor and dentist, in case you need to contact them.

Care Package

Be prepared for minor health problems with a home medical kit. Include brand medications that you know work for you, but that you might not be able to find overseas, like Alka-Seltzer or Advil.

Insure Your Health to Ensure Your Health

It is extremely important for you to have adequate health insurance before departing. Check to see what your policy covers, especially overseas—if you are currently included on your family's insurance policy, you must make sure that the coverage meets your program's insurance requirements and you are covered overseas for the entire time you are there.

What's Up, Doc?

Try to get some information about the health-care system in the region to which you're going. If you need medical care, what will the facilities be like? How do you pay for it? What legal right do you have to medical services? You can get a list of English-speaking doctors worldwide by contacting the International Association for Medical Assistance to Travellers (IAMAT.org).

Money, Money, Money

Only deal with authorized agents when you exchange money, buy airline tickets, purchase souvenirs—keep a small calculator handy to calculate exchange rates. Only use traveler's checks or a credit card (most foreign thieves don't like the hassle and prefer to steal cash).

In Case of Emergency

Have a plan with your family on what you will do in the event of a family emergency, illness, or death. It is much easier to have these conversations before you leave than when you are thousands of miles away and in crisis.[4]

[4] Guidelines © 2010 by Education Dynamics. Reprinted with permission.

A Hostel Environment

Many college students who travel abroad stay in youth hostels, a great and inexpensive option when traveling in a foreign country. However, I do not recommend staying in a hostel by yourself; always have at least one friend with you. If you do plan on staying in hostels, join the Youth Hostel Association in your country, which lets you stay at hostels all over the world. Plan your trip and book ahead, especially if you're going during the summer. The demand for beds is highest during this period, so secure one ahead of time.

While most hostels offer requisite security guarantees, it's advisable to take some basic precautions. Locate the exits, in case of emergency. Don't lose track of your valuables. Exceptionally vital property should be checked with hostel management. Request a receipt—and remember to reclaim your stuff.

Again, the key for traveling abroad is to prepare just like you would in any travel situation. Make smart personal-safety choices, and do your homework on the country where you will be living BEFORE you get there. Respect the customs of the country and learn as much as you can about the culture so when the time comes, you can immerse yourself in the adventure, not worry about staying safe.

How Not to Be an Accidental Tourist

Exploring a new city is a wonderful experience. Finding a fabulous restaurant or cool boutique is always a plus. But your status as a tourist does not have to be tattooed on your forehead. If you have been paying attention to the first part of this chapter, then you already know that the key to being safe is to be *inconspicuous*. This means NO sparkly diamonds, no sassy clothing, and no big wads of money being flashed around. You have your money and traveler's checks safely tucked in your sensible purse and all your valuables are either at home or locked in the hotel safe. Okay, now you're ready to do some sightseeing.

You Can Tell by the Way I Walk . . .

Know where you are going and exactly how to get there. If you need to look at a map, wait until you step into a coffee shop or store to open it up. There is no bigger crime target than the little lost soul, staring at her map dazed and confused in the middle of the sidewalk. When you are walking down the street, act like you know where you are going. Most felons who are interviewed will tell you that they look for the easy targets: those who look scared or unfamiliar with their surroundings. The best defense is *confidence*. When you're out on the street, stand up straight, walk with a purpose, and keep a hand on your purse.

Dress for Success

I'm sure you are a lovely and beautiful young woman, but try not to accentuate your positives by wearing revealing clothing. There is definitely a time and a place for that cute little sundress and those strappy sandals, but your best bet is to dress conservatively with comfortable walking shoes. (I am not suggesting you need to dress frumpy—just don't look like you stepped off the pages of Frederick's of Hollywood, especially if you are traveling alone.) Sex offenders prey on women who are unsure of their surroundings and who are wearing "easily accessible" clothing such as short skirts, dresses, or overalls (the straps are quickly cut with a knife or razor blade).

Mind Your Manners

When you are out in public, be respectful and courteous. Speak in a low, confident tone. There is nothing worse than the loud, rude tourist who is completely oblivious to everyone and everything around her. When I was visiting Germany, I was standing behind an American woman who was trying to change some currency. The polite bank teller began speaking to her in German. The American woman started screaming at her, "Do I look German to you?" and demanded that the teller speak English. People like that make the term "Ugly American" all too real. Be respectful of the city or country that you are visiting.

"Say Cheese!"

I love family photos. My kids cringe when we are visiting somewhere new because I make them pose at every landmark. The fact is it's wonderful to have the memories documented. However, don't get so caught up in getting the perfect shot that you aren't aware of your surroundings. Don't put your purse down while you take the picture of the Eiffel Tower—only to have some crook run by and grab your valuables. Be suspicious of an eager person offering to take the picture for you. You'd be amazed how quickly that "nice" person can disappear with your camera.

Making New Friends

When you are traveling, part of the fun is meeting people. Whether you're with your college friends at a restaurant, or checking out the sights, you don't have to be completely antisocial to be safe. Use your common sense and intuition. If you meet someone, avoid giving the new acquaintance any personal information. Stick to the less personal topics of conversation and whatever you do—DON'T TALK POLITICS (that's always a sure-fire way for violence to erupt). Stay in a very open, public place when socializing with strangers. Never go back to "his place" or to a secluded spot with him—even if the stranger is a babe. If you want to get to know him better, agree to meet for dinner at a crowded restaurant. Do not tell the person where you are staying—give a general response instead like, "I'm staying at a place across town." When you are ready to go home, get in a taxi with the friends you came with—not with a person you just met. If a romance is going to bud, save it for when you get home and can have your new friend checked out first.

Whether you are traveling with college friends or alone, these safety tips will greatly reduce your risk of becoming another "accidental tourist" and you can travel anywhere with confidence and style. That's definitely the Safety Chick way.

Be a Worldly Globe-Trotter

Traveling in other countries requires knowledge of special safety tips you might not be aware of. Julio Mercado is the former deputy director of the U.S. Drug Enforcement Administration (DEA) and current director of security in Latin America and Mexico for the Coca-Cola Company. He has had years of experience teaching people how to stay safe when traveling overseas. He is also a friend of the Safety Chick—so when I asked him what he thought the main security concerns were for college students traveling to other countries, he felt it was important to discuss the possibility of terrorism attacks and kidnap attempts.

Antiterrorism Safety Tips

In today's world, unfortunately, the possibility of terrorism has to be addressed when you travel. While careful security measures are being developed and improved all the time, and while we may hope for a world where it will not be an issue anymore, the fact is terrorism is a highly unlikely but a highly unpredictable danger, so we must be prepared. It is an elusive goal to be able to predict where or when a terrorist act will happen. One of the easiest ways to decrease your odds of becoming a victim is to stay away from areas where there have been persistent terrorist attacks or kidnappings. Julio stresses the importance of once again getting from point A to point B, quickly and safely. For example, do not loiter in airports or train stations. If you need to wait for your transportation or other service, find a place that affords you a good view of the area. If possible, sit with your back against a wall; be a people watcher. If there is an incident, you might have a warning that could permit you to get out or take cover.

- **Be direct**—Book a direct flight into your destination; try to avoid changing airplanes or staying over in high-risk cities.
- **Be a "know nothing"**—Be aware of what strangers might overhear. Keep to yourself where you are from, what your travel plans are, where you are staying. Keep your voice down when talking to friends. In other words: keep a low profile.
- **Don't do crowds**—Avoid public demonstrations or other civil disturbances. Avoid crowded marketplaces and shopping areas.
- **Take note**—Know the location of the U.S. Embassy and other safe locations where you can find refuge or assistance.

Hijacking and Hostage Situations

The current trend in Mexico and some other countries is to kidnap American citizens for ransom. Young American women are easy targets, so you really need to stay on your toes.

While the odds of being kidnapped in a foreign country are slim, the theme of this book and the Safety Chick lifestyle in general is to always think ahead and have a plan. It is important to stay on the main roads and in large cities in countries where kidnapping incidents have occurred. Don't use narrow alleys or dark or poorly-lit streets as shortcuts.

Before you travel abroad, visit www.travel.state.gov and familiarize yourself with the simple guidelines from the U.S. Department of State for hostage situations.

The odds of being in a car accident overseas are much greater than being involved in any terrorist attack or kidnap attempt. Following the information in this chapter allows you to travel the world with confidence. The travel safety and hotel tips should become routine as you travel more and more. Who knows, you might end up with a career that enables you to travel all over the country or even the world!

Safety Chick Checklist:
How to Travel Safely

☒ **BE PREPARED** | Have your travel plans set before you hit the road.

☒ **LEAVE YOUR ITINERARY** | Leave your daily schedule with friends and family back home and check in regularly with them.

☒ **HIT THE GARAGE BEFORE YOU LEAVE** | If you are traveling by car, have a mechanic give it a once-over to make sure everything is in working order.

☒ **TRAVEL IN THE DAY** | Plan your trip so that you are not driving or arriving in a strange city at night.

☒ **TRAVEL IN PACKS** | Remember: safety in numbers—travel with a group of girlfriends and always have each other's backs.

☒ **SPRING BREAK** | Book your trip with a reputable company and get *everything* in writing before you leave.

☒ **FOREIGN TRAVEL** | Check with the Department of State before you leave to find out if there are any current travel warnings in the country you will be visiting, and be sure to register with the American Consulate when you arrive.

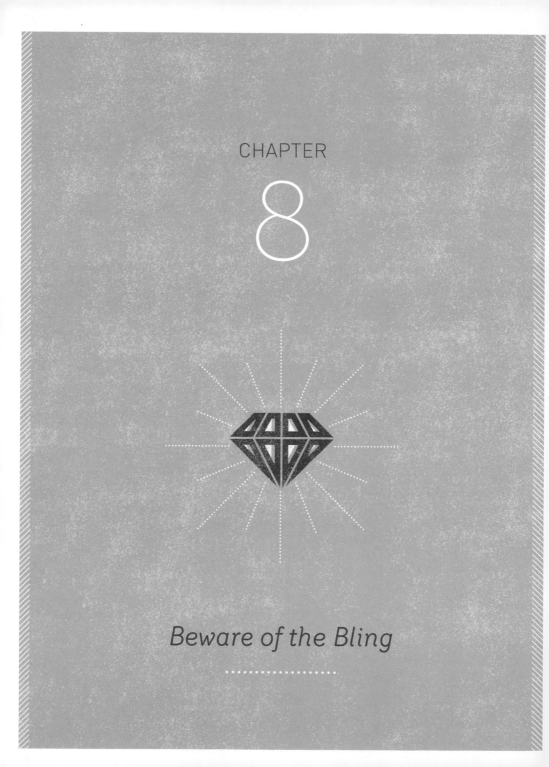

CHAPTER

8

Beware of the Bling

A twenty-three-year-old retail store clerk and Seattle, Washington, college student found herself a victim of identity theft after someone had taken out department store credit cards in her name and racked up thousands of dollars in charges. About a week after a federal agent showed her a picture of the suspect. This young women found herself face-to-face with the woman who stole her identity. The thief had had the bad judgment of attempting to open yet another fraudulent credit account—at the counter of the department store where the victim was the clerk! Fast thinking and level headed, she excused herself and had the store camera zoom in on a fake ID the woman was presenting with another woman's name. This set in motion a federal investigation that ultimately brought down an entire identity theft ring. Federal agents said that without the victim's quick thinking and presence of mind, the take-down would not have been possible.

Being an independent college student also entails financial responsibility. While it might be tempting to open a new credit card to get that cute little dress at the mall to wear on your date Friday night, the downside could be a whole lot more than a lecture from your parents for going over your monthly budget. A large percentage of consumers are in debt by the age of nineteen, and on top of that, college students are at high risk for identity theft. This chapter will give you important info on credit cards and vital tips for staying financially safe.

Watch That Credit

According to Consumers Union, the nonprofit organization that publishes *Consumer Reports*,® credit card companies aggressively market to college students. Why? Because, number one, they see you as fresh meat—someone who has a clean credit record and might be an easy sell. They are banking on the fact that you will spend, spend, spend and not be able to pay off the full amount each month, therefore incurring a penalty that requires you to pay more money to the company. Before you know it, you owe more than you have spent and end up with a whole lot of debt.

Don't get me wrong; credit cards can really help you out financially and aid in building a good credit history, which will be important to you once you are out of school. Having good credit allows you to rent apartments easier, get a loan for a car, or even buy a house. Remember: a financial mistake that you make at eighteen years old will stay on your credit report until you are twenty-five. The key is to understand how to make credit cards work for you—not against you.

Don't ruin your credit before you get out into the real world. Here are some essential tips for every college student applying for and using credit. Doing your research and reading *Consumer Reports*® can give you more in-depth information. Knowing the myths and tips below from Consumers Union is a great start.

1. Myths to Watch for When Signing Up for a Credit Card

A Must-Have in Your Wallet
Credit card companies love to make you think a credit card is indispensable. Think twice before signing up for a credit card you might not need.

Gift with Purchase
What does that free T-shirt or coffee mug really cost? Once you have agreed to the terms set by the credit card company, you may end up paying a lot more for that "free gift" they gave you when you applied for the card. They know how busy students can get, and how easy it is to miss a payment, pay late, or go over your limit. Don't be enticed by a souvenir that may cost you much more in the long run!

"Cancel at Anytime—No Obligations!"
Don't believe it. Many consumers have reported difficulties canceling credit cards they no longer want. Either the customer service representatives were not helpful or they couldn't cancel the card because they carried a balance they could not afford to pay off. Many times those balances were driven up by fees charged on their accounts for the late payments and interest rate hikes. What began as "easy credit" can end up becoming a credit card trap that's difficult to escape.

2. Questions to Ask Yourself Before You Apply

Do I Really Need It?
If you are able to pay for what you need with cash, check, or a debit card, you might not need a credit card. On the other hand, credit cards are great for emergencies and are useful for making secure purchases online. If you already have a credit card, think long and hard about why you would need another one.

Can I Afford It?
If you pay a hefty annual fee just to have a credit card, or regularly carry a balance on your card and pay a high interest rate, you may find yourself spending a lot just to borrow a little. Think about the costs of fees and interest before signing up. On the other hand, you can make your credit card work for you by choosing a card with no annual fee and paying off the balance each month when you get your bill.

What Will I Use It For?
You should never finance your college education or living expenses by using a credit card. Also, using a credit card for things you don't need and can't afford in cash is a bad idea. Sure it's temping to whip out the plastic to buy that bling you have always wanted, but if you are not willing to pay cash for an item, do not buy it on credit. You WILL eventually have to pay for it out of your pocket—plus interest. (If you're not careful, lots and lots of interest, so that in the end you may pay three times the price on that tag you're staring at, or more! Read on.) By charging things you don't need, you'll reach your credit limit quicker and not have the cushion for real emergencies (which is the point of getting the card in the first place!).

How Much Credit Should I Get?
If you are new to credit, or you are a student without a steady income, don't accept a card with a high credit limit just because the credit card issuer is willing to give you one. Sure, it's flattering to be offered a high credit limit, but it might tempt you to charge more than you can realistically pay back. Start out with a low credit limit to test the waters. Also, don't accept an automatic credit limit increase that card issuers often give their cardholders, unless your income has increased sufficiently to pay off more debt.

How Am I Going to Pay for This When the Bill Comes?
If you can pay off your balance every month, you are making the credit card work for you. If you think you are okay because you can make the minimum payment every month, get ready for a very expensive long haul. Though minimum payment amounts can vary among credit cards, one thing is for sure, paying *only* the minimum every month will mean you are paying for years after you leave college—

even if you stop using the card. For example, if you make only the minimum payment due each month on a $1,000 balance, with an 18 percent APR, by some estimates you'll spend seven years and an additional $1,730 in interest to pay back what you owe. By paying only the minimum amount due, you could spend almost twice as long paying off a $1,000 balance as it takes to earn a four-year degree!

3. All Credit Cards Are NOT the Same

Getting into deep credit card debt is a lot easier than you think. But there are some things you can do to make sure you have the upper hand on your credit card situation. Here are some KEY things to look for in the fine print when deciding on a card:

APR
Look for a card with a low APR—this "Annual Percentage Rate" is the interest rate you will pay to borrow money with your credit card. The higher the APR, the more the credit will cost if you don't pay off your balance every month. Watch out for low introductory rates that automatically go up after a set amount of time.

Annual Fee
Look for a card with a low or no annual fee. This is what credit card companies charge you every year, just for having the card. You are obligated to pay this fee. A card with no annual fee and a low interest rate is less expensive.

Changing Terms
Understand the card's "Change of Terms" policy. Many credit card companies reserve the right to change the terms of your credit card agreement at any time and for any reason. This means that the card issuer can raise your interest rate and increase the fees you pay for exceeding your credit limit or paying late. The end result is that the card issuer raises the price you will have to pay on money already borrowed. This is a good reason why it's best to pay off any balance every month. If you don't like the new rules, you can stop using the card.

Universal Default
Look out for something called a "Universal Default" clause. Some credit card companies will raise your interest rate even if you always pay your credit card bill on time and in full. That's because they take into account your bill-paying history with other creditors. Make sure you pay your other bills on time.

4. Be WISE when Using Credit

Pay It Off

Pay off the balance monthly and make your payments on time. If you can't do that, pay off as much as you can afford. Make more than the minimum payment every month.

Keep an Eye on Your Balance

Pay attention to your balance and do not exceed your credit limit. Sometimes the interest charged on a balance or fees you are charged for paying late can put you over your credit limit, which can trigger additional fees.

Don't Take Cash Advances

The interest rate on cash advances is generally higher than the interest rate charged on purchases made with the card. When you make your credit card payments, the card issuer will apply your payments to the lowest interest rate items first, allowing the debt to mount on the higher interest rate items, such as cash advances, until the balance is paid off.

Manage your Account

If you manage your credit card online, be sure to set up e-mail alerts that keep you informed. Many card issuers allow you to set up alerts that tell you when a payment is due, or when you are close to or exceed your credit limit, for example.

5. KISS: Keep It Simple, Student

One Is Enough

If you must have a credit card, one is all you need to build a good credit profile of on-time payments. Besides, having only one card is a good way to avoid credit card confusion when it comes time to pay the bills.

6. If You Get into Trouble, Get Help BEFORE It Gets Out of Hand!

Get Some Guidance

Don't be afraid to ask a family member for help. A little bit of help now can save you a lot of grief in the future. You can also contact a consumer counseling agency in your area to get advice. Learn more at the National Foundation for Credit Counseling's Web site www.nfcc.org (and see Resources on page 195 for more information on credit cards and credit).[5]

[5] Copyright © 2010 by Consumers Union of U.S., Inc., Yonkers, NY 10703-1057, a nonprofit organization. Reprinted with permission from www.consumersunion.org for educational purposes only. No commercial use or reproduction permitted.

How to Stay Safe at the Mall

Now that you have your credit card and are ready to hit the mall, don't forget that there are opportunistic thieves out there who would love to get a hold of your brand-new card. There are important safety tips to follow to make sure criminals don't rip you off.

Keep an Eye on the Prize

Have you ever gone to the grocery store and left your purse in the cart and walked a little farther down the aisle to get something? Have you turned your back in the middle of a sales transaction and left your wallet on the counter to talk on your cell phone or other similar distraction? If you have done anything like that, you are a perfect prey for these lazy thieves. Always keep your purse with you. Many victims are amazed at how quickly their valuables were stolen: "I only looked away for a minute"; "My purse was right next to me a second ago." Don't let this happen to you. If you have to look away or bend over to get something, take your wallet in your hand while you do it.

Home Free

When walking to your car after a successful day of shopping—BE ALERT! I have seen many surveillance videos of victims being robbed of their parcels or having their purses snatched leaving the mall. It is amazing how brazen criminals can be, even in broad daylight. The mistake most of the victims made was that they were completely oblivious to who or what was around them. I watched one bold criminal follow a woman all the way to her car, grab her purse right out of her cart, and jump into a waiting getaway car. The point is, criminals look for the easy target.

Hands Free

If the shoe sale was too good to be true and you have quite a few bags, be sure not to "handcuff" yourself with your purchases. A thief loves a target with her wrist tied up in the handles of her bags, unable to fight as the purse is ripped from her hands. Put your bags in a cart or ask a security guard or mall attendant to help you to your car.

Watch Your Purse

Okay, there are times when your purse can be a fashion statement. But when you are going about your daily life, you really should have a purse that is hard to rip off your body. The best purses are the ones that fit across your body diagonally with thick straps. And remember: Never play tug-of-war with someone who is trying to steal your purse. Let him have it and then scream for the police.

I was driving with my oldest son when we witnessed a young punk on his bike ride by and yank an elderly woman's purse from her shoulder—knocked her right to the ground and broke the strap. The person in the car in front of me was able to block the kid on his bike and I called the police—they arrived shortly thereafter and the woman got her purse back. What struck me was how quickly the whole event occurred and how easily those little purse straps can break. It was also a good lesson for my son to see the young punk taken away in handcuffs. Crime does NOT pay.

If the Worst Happens, Work Fast!

The second you realize that you have been robbed, move into action. First, call the police and file a report. Immediately cancel your credit cards. Experts say that thieves have an approximately two-hour window to use your cards before they are discovered. The sooner you contact the credit card companies, the less damage the thieves can do. The law states that if you report the card stolen before the thief uses it, you cannot be responsible for any unauthorized charges. Make an itemized list of everything that is missing, including credit card numbers, your driver's license number, and any other items, with their monetary value attached. This helps the police with the report and makes it easy for your insurance company to file a claim.

ATM Safety

Recently I did a television segment about ATM skimming. This is when a thief fits a special card reader onto an ATM machine. The slot that now awaits you, the innocent user, looks just like the usual one, but the illegal interface reads the magnetic strip on your card and stores all your information. At the same time, the thief will have concealed a camera somewhere on the machine to record you punching in your PIN. Now the thief not only has your card number, he also has your PIN. It is estimated that close to $1 billion is lost every year to ATM fraud. ADT Security Services just released a device that can be put into the machine and detect if a skimming device has been installed. It shuts down the machine and provides streaming video to the bank of the attempt and, hopefully, pictures of the skimmers themselves.

Remember these three words when using an ATM machine: Observe, Protect, and Ask.

Observe

Look around as you walk up to an ATM—is there anyone lurking in the parking lot? Is the person waiting to use the machine after you standing too close? Pick an ATM that is well lit in a highly trafficked area. Look around or on the machine for any hidden cameras as well. If something seems out of place or doesn't feel right, leave and find another ATM.

Protect

Cover the keypad with your other hand as you punch in your PIN, and use your body to block the screen from "shoulder surfers" (thieves who attempt to stand close to you to try to see your passwords and account information). Take your receipt with you and shred it when you get home. Bottom line: Protect your information.

Ask

Ask your bank if it has an anti-skimming device installed in its ATM machines to guard against skimming.

ID Theft: It Could Happen to You

Identity theft does not just happen to old people with money; I know of a young man named Zach who became a victim when he was seven years old—and he didn't realize it until he was a freshman in college and tried to get a student loan! Due to "poor credit," he not only was turned down for the loan, he also was not hired for a part-time job. He learned that he was forty thousand dollars in debt because someone had bought a houseboat in his name. It took him ten years to attempt to get his credit and good name cleared. While a lot of the damage was fixed, he still has problems from time to time.

In 2008, almost 10 million Americans learned they were victims of identity fraud, up from 8.1 million victims in 2007.

—Javelin Strategy and Research

I was on *The Montel Williams Show* a few years ago with Todd Davis, the founder and CEO of a company called LifeLock, which is dedicated to identity theft protection services. Todd observed that the credit monitoring companies seemed to be reactive rather than proactive when it came to notifying and tracking potential credit fraud. With the number of identity theft victims on the rise, Todd realized the necessity for a service that doesn't just put fraud alerts on your credit card accounts, but is equipped to track your driver's license number, Social Security number, home address, and other vital private and public information when it is being used illegally for credit.

LifeLock also found that college students are at high risk for ID theft. The reason? Student information is out there for the world to see. According to the U.S. Department of Education, almost 50 percent of college students have had grades posted by Social Security number.

Shred It

It is important to have a paper shredder. Many college forms—such as report cards—include personal information that needs to be protected. Unfortunately, an identity thief doesn't need much to steal your identity.
So shred it!

Did you know that it is perfectly legal for someone to go through your trash? In a U.S Supreme Court decision, California vs. Greenwood, they stated that the "expectation of privacy in trash left for collection in an area accessible to the public . . . is unreasonable."

Here is a punch list of items you should shred:

- Address labels from junk mail and magazines
- Any items with a signature (leases, contracts, letters)
- ATM receipts
- Bank statements
- Birth certificate copies
- Cancelled and voided checks

- Credit card bills, carbon copies, summaries, and receipts
- Credit reports and histories
- Documents containing names, addresses, phone numbers, or e-mail addresses
- Documents containing passwords or PIN
- Documents relating to investments
- Employment records
- Expired passports or visas
- Identification cards (college IDs, government IDs, military IDs, employee ID badges)
- Legal documents
- Luggage tags
- Medical and dental records
- Old driver's license or items containing driver's license number
- Papers with a Social Security number
- Pay stubs
- Preapproved credit card applications
- Receipts with checking account numbers
- Report cards
- Resumes or curriculum vitae
- Tax forms
- Transcripts
- Travel itineraries
- Used airline tickets
- Utility bills

Keep Your Personal Info Private—Even from Your Roommate

Dorm, sorority, or apartment living usually means close quarters. Be sure to keep ALL of your personal information and records in a locked, safe-deposit-type box. Do not share your Social Security number, ATM PIN, or other important passwords with anyone, not even your BFF.

Opt Out

Opt out of instant credit applications and other marketing materials that are sent through the mail. Identity thieves can steal these from your mailbox or dig through your trash (if you do not shred), fill them out, and buy a whole new entertainment system on your dime! Call 1-888-5-Opt-Out to get off the list.

Three Major Steps to Stop Telemarketers and the Flow of Junk Mail

1. Contact the three major credit-related organizations

- The Credit Bureau's main opt-out line: (888) 567-8688

This thirty-second call to a computer lets you opt out—meaning they are by law blocked from calling you—of *all* credit-related offers for two years, or permanently.

- Experian Consumer Services: (800) 407-1088

This service removes your name from noncredit offers stemming from Experian lists—the root of (almost) all junk mail evil: samples, coupons, catalogs, and local or national promotional flyers. Again, don't hesitate—it's a thirty-second call to an automated response system.

- Direct Marketing Association (DMA) Opt-Out: www.dma.org

Direct Marketing Association is an industry organization that puts people on a list that is distributed to the more reputable direct mail companies. It puts you on a "do not want to receive" list for national catalogs and marketing companies. There are fees associated when signing up for this service, but if you are one of those inundated with junk mail, organizations like this are a great help. The problem is that many companies don't update their mailing lists for three to six months, so it might take a while before you see any big changes in your junk mail volume.

2. **Mail the list brokers:** These are the companies that sell mailing lists to businesses and organizations. You need to write to them and tell them to take you off all mailing and telemarketing lists.

- Database America
  Compilation Department
  100 Paragon Drive
  Montvale, NJ 07645-0419

- Dunn & Bradstreet
  Customer Service
  899 Eaton Avenue
  Bethlehem, PA 18025

- Metromail Corporation
  List Maintenance
  901 West Bond Street
  Lincoln, NE 68521

- R.L. Polk & Co.—Name Deletion File
  List Compilation Development
  26955 North West Highway
  Southfield, MI 48034

3. **Contact the companies that are currently sending you junk mail:**

- Write to the companies directly requesting to be removed from their lists.
- On postage-paid postcards or enclosed envelopes, write a note telling them to take you off their mailing list. That way you do it on their "dime."
- Call any catalog or junk mail's 800 number and ask them to remove your name and address from their list.
- Write "Refused—Return to Sender" on unopened envelopes you receive that say "address correction requested."

These are somewhat time-consuming steps to take, but well worth it. Junk mail and telemarketing are not only annoying, they are violations of your privacy. Companies that sell your information for personal gain should not be rewarded! Become a "Consumer Assertive" Safety Chick. Don't be afraid to question any person asking you for sensitive information like your Social Security number or your mother's maiden name. First, find out if the information is required or voluntary. If it is voluntary, decline to give it out. If it's required, only give out what is absolutely necessary. Make it clear that you do not want your data available to third parties. If you are not satisfied with their answers do your business elsewhere.

Set Your Fraud Alerts

Setting fraud alerts on all your credit accounts is a must. Do this with all three credit bureaus; they offer this service for free. But remember, fraud alerts don't work if you don't have a credit report. Signing up for a service like LifeLock gives you broader protection that will instantly detect fraudulent use where college students are most vulnerable, especially on the Internet.

Privacy, Please

Your bank, brokerage firms, credit card companies, and insurance companies are required by law to send you a privacy notice each year. Those companies that sell your data to third parties must tell you and give you the chance to opt out. Be sure to make it clear that you do not want your personal information sold. If you have not received a privacy notice, contact the company and have them send you another form.

The most common way an ID thief gets control of a credit card account is via a change-of-address form; the thief simply puts in his address with your name, and he is sent a card. Make sure you assign a "Change of Address alert" to your monitored accounts.

Your Credit Report—Treat It Like Gold

Your credit report holds a great deal of the most personal and vital information you have. The information contained in the report determines crucial decisions made in loans, insurance coverage, employment, even housing. Although according to the federal Fair Credit Reporting Act (FCRA), this information is supposed to remain top secret and extremely confidential, the truth of the matter is, it's relatively easy for anyone to get a hold of these personal records.

Order Your Report

The Federal Trade Commission recommends that you look over a copy of your credit report once a year. To protect yourself even more, you might want to see your report twice a year. A lot of damage can be done in a year—just ask any victims of identity theft. The three biggest credit bureaus are Experian (formerly known as TRW), Equifax, and TransUnion; all you need to do is call or contact them online to receive a copy of your report. You can receive a free report if you have recently been denied credit, have been a victim of fraud, are unemployed, or receive welfare benefits. (See the checklist on page 137 for contact information.)

Steps to Take If You Think You Are a Victim of Identity Theft

There is a list of contact information for all of these organizations at the end of the book. You must work fast and be diligent. Unfortunately, the credit world is not the most effective and organized. It is very easy to get frustrated and give up. The best way to stay on top is to closely read all statements and records, and keep detailed accounts of any problems that arise. It never hurts to fire off a good strong letter to company heads and consumer protection groups—you can let off a little steam and it might just strike a chord with someone who can assist you.

1. **Check your credit report for any new accounts or credit inquires that have shown up; or call immediately if you are sent a "Fraud Alert" (see previous section).**

2. **Contact the credit card company or bank where you have seen inconsistencies or problems with your account.** Ask to speak to the security or fraud department. Review your account with them and highlight any incorrect charges or unauthorized business. If it is more than a billing mistake, you should close the account immediately, and change all ID numbers and passwords.

3. **Contact the major check verification companies if you suspect someone has set up a bank account in your name or is using stolen checks (see Safety Chick Checklist, facing).** If you can pinpoint a merchant that has received one of your stolen checks, find out which verification company they use and contact that company immediately.

4. **Document all contacts.** As with all cases dealing with victimization, you need to be your own detective. In the event of a suspected ID theft, keep a notebook documenting a log of all conversations, complete with names, dates, times of calls, phone numbers, and any other pertinent details.

5. **Contact the fraud department of each of the three major credit bureaus.** Tell them that you think you've been a victim of identity theft and you want them to put a "Fraud Alert" on your file and that no new credit be granted without your approval.

6. **File a police report.** Get a copy of the report for the bank, credit card company, or anyone else who might need proof that a crime was committed.

7. **File a complaint with the Federal Trade Commission (FTC) hotline:** The FTC doesn't actually deal with the prosecution of identity theft, but it can help victims resolve financial problems that can occur as a result of the theft.

8. **Contact the U.S. Postal Inspection Service** if you think a criminal has submitted a change of address in your name or used any other postal service to commit acts of fraud.

9. **Contact the U.S. Social Security Administration** if you think your Social Security number is being fraudulently used.

10. **Contact the Internal Revenue Service** if you think improper use of your identity has interfered with tax violations.

About 62 million trees and 25 billion gallons of water are used to produce a typical year's worth of junk mail in the United States.

—Fightidentitytheft.com

Safety Chick Checklist:
What to Do If You're a Victim of Fraud

IF CREDIT CARDS ARE STOLEN:
☒ Contact all of your credit card companies IMMEDIATELY to report stolen cards.

☒ Put a "Fraud Alert" on all accounts.

☒ File a report with local police.

IF YOU ARE A VICTIM OF IDENTITY THEFT:
☒ Get a copy of your credit report.

☒ File a police report.

☒ File a report with the Federal Trade Commission: (877) 438-4338.

☒ Contact the three major credit bureaus (Fraud Department): Experian: (888) 397-3742; Equifax: (800) 525-6285; TransUnion: (800) 680-7289.

☒ Contact all creditors with whom you have found evidence of fraudulent charges on bills.

☒ Contact all financial institutions where you have accounts.

☒ Contact major check verification companies (Fraud Department): Check Rite: (800) 766-2748; ChexSystems: (800) 428-9623; CrossCheck: (800) 552-1900; Equifax: (800) 437-5120; TeleCheck: (800) 710-9898.

☒ Contact the Social Security Administration: (800) 269-0271.

☒ Contact the Internal Revenue Service: (800) 829-0433.

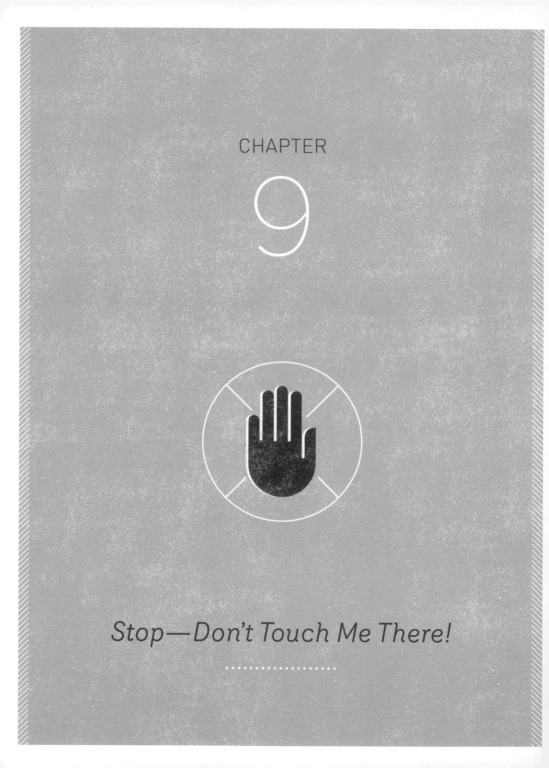

CHAPTER

9

Stop—Don't Touch Me There!

When I was an undergrad at UCLA, my girl-friends and I decided to take a history class together one quarter. We had all heard that it was an easy class. The rumor was that the professor was an old guy who had been teaching there for years and liked young girls. If he liked you, he gave you an A without you having to do much work. We all decided we could use a break from our heavy schedules, so we signed up. Turned out, the rumors were true.

One day I stayed after class to talk to my professor about the fact that I was going to miss an exam he had scheduled for the following week. After everyone had left the classroom, he pulled me down on his lap and had me talk to him from there. He said I was a cute girl with a lot of personality and he liked having me in his class. Words cannot describe how incredibly awkward, embarrassed, and uncomfortable I felt at that moment. I had no idea how to get out of the situation. There were so many thoughts rushing through my mind . . . is this guy who is older than my father hitting on me, or is he just trying to be nice and nurturing, like my grandpa? If I get up and walk out, will he give me an F? If I sit here and smile, will I get an A? After a few agonizing moments, he let me up with a little squeeze and a pat on the butt. I left his classroom shaken and very angry. I talked to my friends about it and a few of them said they had had similar experiences with him. But none of us ever did anything about it. We just made sure never to be alone with him again. By the way—we all got As.

Entitlement and Title IX

To understand the concept of sexual harassment and discrimination of women, it is helpful to learn about the roots from which the current laws that protect us stem. Discrimination toward the female gender has been around for a long, long time. Heck, less than a century ago, women were not allowed to *vote*!

Even the climate on supposedly enlightened college campuses was also very much a man's world until pretty recently. Programs and activities on campuses were not equally available to woman, and inequalities in grading, employment, salaries, and other measures of accomplishment were extremely prevalent. The term "sexual harassment" did not yet exist, and a woman who was strong and independent was, in many cases, not received well. If not for those very strong and independent women years ago, the wonderful opportunities to which you, the young women of today growing into your roles as leaders and doers of tomorrow, are entitled would not exist. These are the women behind Title IX.

Title IX: "No person in the United States shall, on the basis of sex, be excluded from participation in, be denied the benefits of, or be subjected to discrimination under any education program or activity receiving Federal financial assistance."

The Godmother of Title IX

Dr. Bernice R. Sandler is a senior scholar at the Women's Research and Education Institute in Washington, DC, where she consults with institutions and others about achieving equity for women. She played a major role in the development and passage of Title IX in 1972, along with other laws prohibiting sexual discrimination in education, and has been associated with Title IX longer than any other person. She is well known for her expertise in women's educational equity in general as well as in sexual harassment, the chilly classroom climate, and policies, programs, and strategies concerning women on campus. She also serves as an expert witness in discrimination and sexual harassment legal cases.

Dr. Sandler is one strong and brave chick. As I stated in the introduction to this book, what you as young women must understand is that no matter what stage of life you are in, we are all in this together. No matter how old or young, women are the number one victims of crime, and it takes women like you, me, Dr. Sandler, and all the other courageous champions—those mentioned in this book and the countless others around the globe—to truly make a difference and make our lives safe from crime. I recommend that you read Dr. Sandler's fascinating story, available on her Web site, www.bernicesandler.com, to better understand how her strength and integrity dramatically changed the lives of women.

What Is Sexual Harassment?

According to the U.S. Equal Employment Opportunity Commission (EEOC), sexual harassment is defined as "unwelcome sexual advances, requests for sexual favors, or other verbal or physical conduct of a sexual nature." Same-sex harassment is also prohibited.

What actually constitutes sexually harassing behavior is a bit harder to define, because it encompasses such a broad range of actions. To begin understanding how to recognize sexual harassment, here is a partial list of behavior types:

- **Gender harassment**—includes statements and behavior that convey insulting, degrading, and/or sexist attitudes.
- **Seductive behavior**—encompasses unwanted, inappropriate, and/or offensive physical or verbal sexual advances.
- **Sexual bribery**—involves the solicitation of sexual activity or other sex-linked behavior by threat of punishment or promise of reward.
- **Sexual assault**—attempted rape and rape.

For the purposes of our discussion, we can say that, basically, sexual harassment falls into two categories: verbal and physical. In terms of verbal, it can be as simple as that clichéd image—and it still happens—of a woman walking by a construction site and all the workers whistling at her and making rude comments like, "Hey baby—looking good today." Another example, perhaps more clouded by power roles, could be a male boss saying to his female coworker, "Gee Julie, that blouse makes your boobs look really big." Some verbal harassment might be more discreet, like the male student sitting next to you in science class who is always talking about sexual things: "I had such a crazy night last night, hooked up with two girls at once . . . do you like that sort of thing?" or "I love porn movies, saw a great one last night." Bottom line is: any innuendos or comments of a sexual nature that make you feel uncomfortable, angry, hurt, or embarrassed are indeed sexual harassment.

Physical sexual harassment is a little easier to identify, although certainly no easier to take. Inappropriate touching (like when my professor pulled me down on his lap and then patted my rear end as I stood up) constitutes physical sexual harassment. Or, for example, if another student repeatedly brushes against you, pretending to sharpen his pencil or what have you, even if not near what we think of as private areas, like breasts and rear end—that's physical sexual harassment. More obvious behavior is, of course, if you are unwillingly kissed or fondled by someone. Bottom line again: you are the boss of your body—no one may touch you in an inappropriate or unwanted manner.

Dealing with Sexual Harassment

Many people who experience sexual harassment and feel uncomfortable may not initially recognize the behavior as sexual harassment. Often there is a tendency on the part of the person who experienced the behavior to minimize or deny its meaning by saying "I'm sure he didn't really mean it," or "It's really no big deal," or "I must be imagining this"—first to herself and perhaps then to others she may tell about it. Sometimes if the harasser is a respected person, someone in authority, or a close friend, denial and shock may set in so that the person who is harassed is simply unable to deal with the incident(s) for several days or weeks, or ever.

Protecting yourself against sexual harassment is no different than any other personal-safety issue in this book. While how you choose to deal with sexual harassment is up to you, here are some of Bernice Sandler's great ideas for responses and reactions to sexually harassing behavior:

The "Miss Manners" Approach

"I beg your pardon!" This protest, coupled with strong facial expressions of shock, dismay, and disgust can be used whenever you cannot think of anything else to say or do. A variant of this is "I can't believe you actually said that!" or "I'm speechless!"

The "Ball Buster" Approach: Naming or Describing the Behavior

"That comment is offensive to women; it is unprofessional and is probably sexual harassment. That behavior has to stop." Or, "This is the third time you have put your arm around me. I don't like it and I don't want you to do that anymore."

The Me "No Comprende" Approach: Pretending Not to Understand

This is particularly useful with sexist or sexual remarks and jokes. You keep a deadpan expression and state that you don't get the point or don't understand what this means. Follow up by asking the person to repeat whatever it is he just said, and again claim that you don't understand what he means. There is nothing worse for a joke teller or someone who thinks he or she has made a clever remark than to be told that someone didn't "get it." After you do this two or three times, the person or someone else may explain what the remark means or why it is supposed to be funny. If not, you can ask the person to explain it to you. In either event, you silently wait for a few seconds and then simply say, "Oh." Hopefully, the other person will understand that the behavior is inappropriate, but even if the "joker" (that is, offender) does not, he or she may not make these remarks to you anymore, believing that you have no sense of humor or because you are not responding to the "jokes" in the way the speaker wanted.

The "You Must Be a Comedian" Approach: Using Humor

Because they connote strength, humor and playfulness are good ways to handle these issues if you can think of something immediately. They are ways of saying that the comment didn't get to you and did not accomplish what the speaker wanted it to, which typically is to make you uncomfortable. Unfortunately, many of us think of wonderful funny remarks later, when they aren't needed. However, here are some standard responses, which, said lightly and jokingly, might be useful:

"Uh-oh—that is sexual harassment—you had better watch out before you get in big trouble."

"Are you sexually harassing me again? I am going to have to call the sexual harassment committee (my attorney, Gloria Allred, the affirmative action officer, etc.) right now.

Practice these responses in front of a mirror to get more comfortable with them. Sometimes in an attempt to cope with sexually harassing remarks, women may giggle at the harasser's behavior, joke back, or initiate a sexual discussion. This behavior is rarely successful in stopping sexual harassment because the harasser does not recognize that the behavior is not welcomed by the woman and thus he continues the behavior.

Would You Like to Be in My Book? The "Sexual Harassment Notebook"

Buy a notebook and write in bold letters on the cover "Sexual Harassment." When the behavior happens, take out the notebook and casually state "Could you say that again? I want to write it down." Make a big show of asking for the date, the time, noting your exact location, etc. If asked why you are writing things down, you can blandly say, "I'm just writing things down" or "I'm thinking of writing a book about sexual harassment."

The Sexual Harassment Research Project

This variant of the Sexual Harassment Notebook is also particularly helpful in dealing with recurrent sexual harassment, including harassment by a group. Upon hearing a degrading remark, whip out a copy of a "project form" and say, "I'm so glad you said that. I'm doing research on sexual harassment. Would you mind if I ask you some questions?" The piece of paper you are armed with is filled with questions about sexual harassment, such as "How often do you do this?" "How do you choose people to harass?" "Do you discuss this with your girlfriend or your mother?" "Would you act like this if a person's significant other were present?" You can make up questions like this. If someone asks for whom you are doing your research, you have permission to use Bernice Sandler's name!

The Letter

This technique, developed by Mary Rowe at the Massachusetts Institute of Technology, has been extraordinarily successful in dealing with sexual harassment and other forms of interpersonal conflict. The letter consists of three parts.

Part I:
Describe what happened in a very factual manner, without any evaluative or judgmental words, such as, "Last week you called me a 'bitch' and a 'whore.'" Usually people agree about the facts but disagree about the interpretation of those facts. What this section of the letter does is separate the facts from the feelings.

Part II:
Describe how you feel about the incident(s), again without evaluating the perpetrator, such as, "I am really uncomfortable with this behavior. I find it offensive." Or "When I am around you, I feel physically ill."

Part III:
This part is generally very short, describing what you want to have happen next. "I want the behavior to stop" or "I want to be treated in a professional manner, the way every student has a right to be treated."

Send the letter by certified mail with a return receipt requested, as a way of impressing upon the recipient that it is important. Sending the letter by certified mail provides the writer with evidence that the letter was received. Should the harassment continue, the letter can be used as evidence that sexual harassment existed and, along with the receipt, shows that you took steps to inform the perpetrator that the behavior was unwelcome.

Keep a copy of the letter, but do not send a copy of it to anyone else. If, for example, the letter said "cc: the Dean," the recipient of the letter might charge into the dean's office in an attempt to destroy your credibility. The letter works best if it is a private communication between two individuals.

The letter is successful 90 to 95 percent of the time. It will not work with a very hostile person or someone who is sadistic or with groups of harassers. Most of the time, the harasser says nothing but stops the behavior. Once in a while, the harasser wants to apologize or explain, but it is best not to get into a discussion of the behavior. Simply say, "I'm not going to discuss it. I just want the behavior to stop."[6]

What to Do If Your Professor Makes an Unwanted Move

It's bad enough if the guy in your math class keeps making unwanted sexual advances, but if the inappropriate behavior is coming from your professor or someone in a position of authority, things can become very complicated. There are some instances where you really hit it off with a professor. He might just see you as a really smart and creative student, or he might go above and beyond for you because he sees something in you that he sees in himself; a special intellectual connection with a teacher is one of the most rewarding things in higher education. However, true and responsible educators will never overstep the boundary between the student-teacher relationship and the personal, and absolutely NEVER is it acceptable to apply even the most indirect or subtle sexual advances toward you. If you recognize that flattery—telling you that you are the best student in class or of his career, for example—or pressure—such as inviting you to use sexual favors in exchange for

[6] Responses to Sexual Harassing Behavior reprinted with permission of Bernice Sandler, www.bernicesandler.com.

better grades—is coming from a teacher or administrator, it is important to do something about it. Reporting the incident is one way to protect yourself, and also to protect other students from suffering the same fate.

Reporting Sexual Harassment

If you have a truly aggressive sexual harasser, much like a stalker, you need to take serious action to end this abuse against you. Start documenting the perpetrator's behavior, and take steps to organize a complaint against him. If you feel the situation warrants it, you can start with informal complaints through the support systems of your school. Read Chapter 10 thoroughly, as well as the next section, which was written in collaboration with Bernice Sandler, for information on how to document and where to get the support you need to make a complaint or a formal charge.

Keep a Diary

Keep a diary or some sort of record if sexual harassment happens more than once, or if you experience a situation that feels seriously inappropriate or has led to unwanted physical contact of any kind. Write down the date, time and place, witnesses, what happened, and what your response was. Many months later, it might be important to remember these details. You need to have the incident and the details straight if you decide to file a formal complaint with the authorities.

Share with Others

You probably aren't the only person who is being harassed by this person. (Remember my professor?) Virtually all harassers are serial harassers; their behavior with you is most likely not an isolated incident . . . talk to other women.

Get the Paperwork

Go to your women's health center, dean's office, or student affairs office and get copies of any materials your university has on sexual harassment. Talk to your dean or other senior administrator, and begin to educate yourself as well. Become familiar with the school's policies and procedures for dealing with harassment, and then decide if or how you would like to proceed. Take notes as you talk or write down what was said after the meeting.

Send Him a Message

If you think it's appropriate, send a copy of the school's Sexual Harassment Policy to the person who is making you uncomfortable. If you don't want to send it under your name, oftentimes a women's group will send it, along with a note saying that they thought it would be of interest to the recipient.

Don't Deal with Stress Alone

Just like any other victimization, being sexually harassed can cause stress, fear, and anger. Seek counseling from your women's health center or a professional psychologist for help on coping.

Put It in Writing

If none of the informal methods have worked to stop the harassment, you should consider filing a formal complaint. Generally, you should do this with your school; however, if you feel the persons in charge are not responding properly, you might need to file charges outside of the institution, either with the appropriate governmental agency or through the courts.

Domestic Violence: It Doesn't Just Happen on an Episode of *COPS*

One night I was home from college having dinner with my parents and my older brother. The house was on a corner of a relatively busy street. We were startled by the sound of a young woman screaming. By the time my brother and I ran outside, the woman was being thrown out of a slow-moving pickup truck. Thankfully, she landed in the ivy along the road. When we got to her, she was huddled up in a ball, crying. My brother touched her shoulder and when she looked up, we were shocked to see that it was a childhood friend of mine, whom I knew quite well. She immediately blurted, "Don't call my parents . . . my Dad will kill him." She was talking about her boyfriend—the man who had just thrown her out of his truck. They continued to have a very tumultuous relationship, and she continued to get knocked around. Somehow, I just didn't quite get the romance and excitement of being thrown from a moving vehicle.

Domestic violence is an epidemic in this country. Thankfully, the laws are starting to get really tough on the offenders. As women, we need to take responsibility as well. Learning to identify abusive behavior before you get into a situation you can't get out of is a great place to start. Our country is a world leader in cutting-edge programs, shelters, and organizations for women who are victims of domestic violence. But in order to get help, you need to understand the definition of domestic violence and how to recognize signs and behaviors of victimization.

One of the best educational organizations in the area of domestic abuse is the National Coalition Against Domestic Violence. (See Resources, page 195, for how to reach them.) They have worked to provide clear definitions of what battering is and the different forms it takes to help you recognize when to say no.

Hey Batterer, Batterer, Batterer

Domestic abuse can take many forms. It may include emotional abuse, economic abuse, and/or sexual abuse. Tactics include threats, intimidation, and other power plays. Women are the most common victims of this violence, but elder and child abuse also is tragically prevalent.

Battering is a way for a person to establish power or control over another person through fear and intimidation. This can include the threat or use of violence. The batterer (or abuser) believes that he is entitled to control another person. Battering, like assault, is domestic violence; both of these are crimes.

TIP #1 Love Means Never Having to Say, "I'm Sorry I Punched You in the Eye" and Other Lessons in Recognizing Domestic Abuse

Categories of Domestic Abuse

- **Physical Battering**—The abuser's physical attacks or aggressive behavior can range from bruising to murder. It often begins with what are excused as trivial incidents, then escalates into more frequent and serious attacks.
- **Sexual Abuse**—Physical attack by the abuser often is accompanied by, or culminates in, sexual violence, wherein the woman is forced to have sexual intercourse with her abuser or take part in unwanted sexual activity.
- **Psychological Battering**—The abuser's psychological or mental violence can include constant verbal abuse, harassment, excessive possessiveness, isolating the woman from friends and family, deprivation of physical and economic resources, and destruction of personal property.

The most important thing to remember about battering is: It escalates. It often starts with behavior like name calling, violence in the victim's presence (like punching a fist through a wall in anger), and/or damaging objects or pets. It may then turn to restraining, pushing, slapping, and/or pinching. The batterer might begin to punch, kick, bite, or trip. Sexual assault and throwing the victim around might come into play next. Finally, the behavior may become life-threatening—choking, breaking bones, or using weapons. This escalation is very dangerous and any pattern resembling the one described above must be taken very seriously—remember, it may start as just the calling of names.

Red Flags for Domestic Abuse

A number of behavioral signs, often occurring before actual abuse, are typical of domestic abusers. These can serve as warnings. If you are dating someone who is making you feel unsafe in any way, or who is outright threatening or violent, ask yourself these questions to help assess the situation and see the signs before it is too late.

- **Did he grow up in a violent family?** People who have been abused as children or who grew up in a home where one parent beat another may have learned to feel that violence is normal behavior.

- **Does he tend to use force or violence to solve his problems?** A guy who gets into fights, likes to talk tough, and/or has a quick temper is likely to act that way toward his girlfriend. Does he punch or throw things when he gets upset? Does he overreact to problems or frustration? Is he violent toward animals? Does he have a criminal record? (That one is obviously a glaring beacon of warning.) Any or all of these may signal that he is a person who resolves dissatisfaction or aggravation with violence.

- **Does he abuse alcohol or other drugs?** There is a strong link between violence and problems with drugs and alcohol. If he refuses to admit or accept that he has a drug dependency or alcohol problem and refuses to get help, DO NOT think you can change him.

- **Does he have strong traditional ideas about what a man should be and what a woman should be?** Look, this isn't the 1950s anymore; a relationship should be like a partnership, not a dictatorship. Does he think you should stay home instead of going out with your girlfriends? Does he text you every minute demanding to know where you are and what you are doing? Does he put you down if you express your ideas or concerns? Do you feel like a prisoner in your relationship? This mindset leads to dysfunction and destruction.

- **Is he jealous of your other relationships?** This applies not just to other men that you may know, but also to your relationships with your women friends and your family. Does he keep tabs on you? Does he want to know where you are at all times? Does he not let you socialize with your friends without him coming along? Does he isolate you at his side constantly? Remember: *Possessiveness leads to aggressiveness.*
- **Does he have access to guns, knives, or other lethal instruments?** Does he have a fascination with guns or other types of weapons? While this may seem to fit into a normal passion for movies or video games, anything beyond a hobbyist attitude is reason for caution. Does he threaten to use weapons against people to get even? Walk away from this at once.
- **Does he expect you to follow his orders or read his mind?** Does he become unusually angry if you do not fulfill his every wish, or if you cannot anticipate his every want and need? You are not his *I Dream of Jeannie*; no healthy relationship asks this of a partner.
- **Does he go through extreme highs and lows?** This behavior, called "manic," can seem as if he's almost two different people—really sweet and kind at one time, and extremely cruel or violent at another. It may be a sign that he needs counseling or other medical attention for his mental health—and this is not your job.
- **When he gets angry, do you fear him?** Do you find that you feel as if you are walking on eggshells around him? Do you always do what he wants you to do rather than what you want to do? Does a major part of your life revolve around not making him angry?
- **Does he treat you roughly?** Is he physical with you if you do not do what he wants? Does he lash out at you if he is frustrated? Shoving is considered rough treatment; pushing or kicking is a higher level of bad. Do NOT tolerate any such treatment.

If the guy you're involved with exhibits any of these traits, reconsider the relationship before it goes any further. **If he is guilty of several, you should end all contact with him at once.** *It's up to you to set standards for yourself.* While the wild, bad boys might be attractive and sexy in Hollywood movies, in the real world they lead to nothing but trouble and heartache. Set higher expectations for men whom you have relationships with, and you'll be surprised at the number of nice guys you'll attract.

"A friend can tell you things you don't want to tell yourself."

—Frances Ward Weller

If the Shoe Fits

Batterers come from all different backgrounds and with many different personalities. But there are general characteristics that fit the profile of most batterers; be alert for these.

- **Oink, oink**—Batterers are basically male chauvinist pigs who do not see women as people, but as property or sexual objects. They do not respect women as a group.
- **Mr. Insecurity**—The typical batterer suffers from low self-esteem; a sense of powerlessness and ineffectiveness in the world is his inner secret. He may appear to be successful, but inside he feels extremely inadequate.
- **It's all your fault**—Batterers blame other people for their problems or behavior. Stress, something his partner did, alcohol, or other factors become the batterer's excuse for his violent reactions.
- **A big phony**—The batterer often is seen as charming and sweet by the neighborhood, but behind closed doors, it's another story. He can be calm and loving to his partner one time and extremely volatile the next.
- **You belong to me**—Character traits of potential batterers include extreme jealousy, possessiveness, and a bad temper. If a guy is unpredictable and/or verbally abusive, find another date.

Domestic violence happens in rich neighborhoods and poor neighborhoods. Batterers come in all ages, skin colors, and nationalities. It is their behaviors— some subtle characteristics, some socially "excused," some frightening and disorienting—that set them apart from other men.

Why Stay When There is a Way Out

TIP #2 R-E-S-P-E-C-T, Find Out What It Means to Me—Understanding Why and How to Gain the Strength to Get Out of an Abusive Relationship

If you are in an abusive relationship, you need to get the heck out. Life is too short to be with someone who treats you badly. It might seem too scary and overwhelming to contemplate leaving, but for your safety, you need to do it. You might be asking yourself, "Why does he treat me like this? I know deep down inside he loves me." So, to help you understand why men batter women, I will draw again on the great wisdom of the National Coalition Against Domestic Violence (NCADV).

According to the NCADV, there are many speculations on why men batter their mates. The batterer begins and then continues the behavior because he believes that violence is an effective method for gaining and keeping control over another person. Plus, he usually does not suffer any adverse consequences as a result of his behavior. Historically, domestic violence has never really been treated as a real crime. Among the evidence that supports this is a low rate of incarceration or financial penalties for men guilty of abusing their partners. These guys are likely to escape being ostracized by their peer groups or communities, even if it is known that they beat their partners. Therefore, people who are quite literally guilty feel no guilt or sense of wrongdoing.

Regardless of the reason, many women stay in these violent, dangerous relationships when they need to get out, possibly to save their lives. With education and strong support, more and more women are finding the strength to do so. If you are one of these women, there are many places that you can go to for help. Programs like the Office of Violence Against Women through the U.S. Department of Justice and the National Coalition Against Domestic Violence have wonderful support groups and services to assist you in your time of need. Just call their 800 numbers or go to their Web sites for more information. Refer to the Resources section at the end of the book for more information and help near you.

TIP #3 READY, SET, GO—How to Make a Plan to Remove Yourself from a Harmful Situation and Get to Safety

"It's important that people should know what you stand for. It's equally important that they know what you won't stand for." **—Mary H. Waldrip**

If you realize that you have gotten yourself into a violent relationship, there are vital steps to follow to get out and get safe. Read carefully and take heart. There are three vital steps for getting out.

1. Prior to a Violent Incident

- Make plans to leave before violence occurs. Learn how to identify the level of violence your boyfriend (or any male friend or relative) is capable of, so that you can assess danger to yourself. For example, most batterers have a cycle of violence, exhibiting it when they are stressed out at school, if something has upset them, or if they have been drinking or abusing drugs. Become aware of what sets off your abuser and steer clear of all things in this category until you can complete a safe break from the relationship.

- Make arrangements with a trusted friend, or a friend of a trusted friend whom your boyfriend *does not know* to help you. Go to a safe place, such as a friend's home or a domestic violence shelter, and expect to stay there until you and your support system can evaluate that his reaction will not be a danger to you. Ask her not to tell anyone that she is helping you.

- Know your local battered women's shelter phone number.

- Plan where you will go in an emergency or if the situation does become dangerous (e.g., a shelter or safe family member's home).

- If you believe your boyfriend may come to your classroom or workplace, instruct your teacher or employer not to talk with him. Have them notify you if he shows up and wants to speak with you and then call 911.

2. During a Violent Incident

- Leave the physical presence of the batterer, if possible.

- Leave the area or get to a room with a lock on the door and/or a phone.

- If you have a phone, call 911, then call your local shelter for battered women.

- If you do not have a phone, and even if you do, scream so your neighbors can hear; they may call the police or come to your aid.

- If you cannot get out of the violent situation, defend yourself to the best of your ability (see Chapter 11).

3. A Safe Escape

If you find yourself in a situation where you fear you may need to leave campus immediately to feel safe, put a few things in an "escape bag": money, an extra set of keys, a change of clothes, important documents, and phone numbers. Bottom line: Escape to safety—if you have time to assemble them, these few things may arm you to feel calm, focused, and prepared. If you are in immediate danger, however, do not wait around to pack.

Domestic violence is a complicated issue. Talk to your women's health center or a local shelter or victim assistance office to get more information on how to manage your personal situation. (See Resources, page 195, for more information.) Remember: *There is always a way to get out of an abusive relationship.* A young, smart college student deserves better, and you owe it to yourself. Be strong, have courage, and use the wisdom of the domestic violence shelters and law enforcement agencies that are there to help you. Safety Chicks everywhere are behind you.

Dating and being in a committed relationship are difficult enough; the sooner you understand how to deal with and protect against aggressive members of the opposite sex, the healthier relationships you will have. Whether it's sexual harassment or domestic violence, standing up for yourself and handling the situation makes you a stronger Safety Chick. As I once said on *The Montel Williams Show* in a discussion of domestic violence: "There are a lot of fish in the sea . . . hold out for a good one."

Safety Chick Checklist:
What to Do If You Are Being Sexually Harassed

✖ **PLAN** | Pick a strategy that suits you and the situation.

✖ **REACT** | If the behavior doesn't stop, consider writing a letter to the harasser.

IF HE STILL WON'T GIVE IT A REST:

✖ Document and safe-keep all evidence.

✖ Report behavior to school officials such as the staff at the Women's Health Department, the dean, officers of student affairs, etc.

✖ File a formal complaint with the campus police, the Department of Justice, the offices of Violence Against Women, etc.

CHAPTER

10

*I'll Follow You
Until You Love Me*

One day, a beautiful and talented college student started receiving weird e-mails from a guy she had gone to high school with. He was not a close friend of hers, but had been in her photography class a few years before. In that class, he often took pictures of her and posted them various places around campus. During her freshman year at college, his e-mails started, as well as calls to her parents at home to find out when she was coming to visit. Once, he even called her sorority house to attempt to speak with her. Thinking the behavior was strange, her father decided to call his parents, and when he spoke with them he got some disturbing information. It turned out the boy was suffering from schizophrenia and depression. He had been kicked out of school and could not hold a job. This quick-thinking father immediately contacted his daughter's campus police to let them know what had been going on. Over the Christmas break, she drove home with her mother. Around the same time, the boy's family went to his apartment and found the front door wide open, the TV on, and some of his clothes missing. They notified the authorities. A few days later, the police discovered a young man who was camped out in her dorm lounge on campus. It was her high school acquaintance, looking for her. Lucky for her, she was safe with her parents at home.

The Definition of the Crime of Stalking

I cannot tell you how many times I have heard the argument from guys over the years, "Jeez, all I was trying to do was ask the girl out . . . you know how girls say 'no' when they really mean 'yes'?" Or maybe, "If I had taken 'no' for an answer, my wife and I wouldn't be married today!" When we were first trying to get the anti-stalking law passed in every state, I went on several television and radio shows. I always met the same argument, either from defense attorneys, ACLU members, or just men in general. None of them seemed to get the fact that the crime of stalking was a whole lot more than an innocent guy trying to woo a girl into courtship. Many people identify the crime of stalking with celebrities. It's true that Madonna, Brad Pitt, and Tyra Banks all have been victims, but the reality is that stalking is a crime that can touch anyone.

"Every step you take—every move you make—I'll be watching you."

—Sting, "Every Breath You Take"

A stalker is defined by the California Penal Code as "any person who willfully, maliciously, and repeatedly follows or harasses another person and who makes a credible threat with the intent to place that person in reasonable fear for his or her safety." (To find a definition of the Stalking Law in your state, check with your Attorney General's office.) We have come a long way legally since the crime of stalking was first given a name.

Unfortunately, many people still have a difficult time recognizing that this dangerous criminal act is serious. It took me a while to realize that my situation was threatening. We as women are so used to men making unwanted advances, we sometimes go numb to their persistence. I know that I kept thinking the man who was stalking me was going to stop. After he was arrested with 180 rounds of ammunition and a semiautomatic weapon and told the police he wanted to kidnap me, I finally came to the realization that this was more than a little crush. Do not let denial replace good common sense. Recognizing early signals of stalking can be the key to preventing a dangerous situation.

Can't This Guy Take a Hint? How to Recognize Stalking Behavior

How can you tell if you are being stalked or you're just the focus of a guy who is into you and a little slow getting the message? The first step is to think about how you know the person and use your intuition to assess the situation.

The Acquaintance

A lot of times, stalkers who are acquaintances will misconstrue what you are telling them and twist it to mean that you are interested. For example, the guy at

Jamba Juice who makes your smoothie every Tuesday morning when you come in after yoga class finally gets up the guts to ask you out. You tell him, "Thank you, but I'm in a relationship." What he hears in his delusional mind is: "Gee, I would really like to go out with you, but I've got this darned boyfriend. Maybe we can work something out." He now begins a relentless campaign to get you to go out with him. Maybe he starts following you around town, parking in front of your dorm to see you, or making harassing phone calls. This is stalking behavior.

The Nightmare Date from Hell

Let's be honest, we've all had a few of these. Your friend has a friend whose brother's roommate has a cousin who would be perfect for you. You meet him for dinner. Somewhere between the appetizer and dessert, you realize his elevator doesn't quite go to the top. You make it to the end of the night when he says, "Gee, I had a wonderful time, when can we get together again?" You, being the polite, courteous young woman that you were groomed to be, lie and say, "Well, thank you, but I'm swamped with school work right now, I'll have to let you know." Then you spend the next week screening your calls. In most cases, the guy will get the hint. Unfortunately, it can also be the precise catalyst that prompts a stalker. Suddenly you start receiving unwanted flowers or gifts from the guy. He starts showing up outside your English class. If he won't leave you alone, it is stalking behavior.

The Ex

In the immortal words of Usher, "Gotta let it BURN . . .," meaning, let go of a past relationship. But sometimes, people just can't let go. In many countries, it is absolutely unacceptable for the woman to leave the man. Doing so can lead to death. And the truth is that even in America, some guys have difficulty dealing with separation as well. Rejection is not an option they accept, and it can lead to intense harassment or physical violence. For example, maybe you have broken up with your boyfriend and are dating someone else. And your ex-boyfriend gets extremely angry and starts making threatening phone calls to both of you. Maybe he starts showing up in front of your house at all hours of the night. Even if he was not abusive toward you when you were together, be careful. You never know what is going to trigger stalking behavior. Depression, drug use, or extreme stress all can be contributing factors. Whatever the reason might be, even if these actions seem out of character, there is NO excuse for this kind of stalking behavior.

The Lab Partner

This can be similar to the acquaintance scenario, but the difference is that you see this person every day. He could be the guy in science class or on your club sports team. The problem comes when he starts making unwanted advances. Because you are forced to be in the same place as him every day, you can't get away from him. He might start leaving notes on your desk or send unwanted e-mails. He may even become more aggressive in front of other students. For example, you already have rejected his e-mail inviting you to dinner days before. He approaches you before class and loudly says, "Why haven't you returned any of my phone calls? I really thought we had something going here!" (which in and of itself is bizarre, considering you have never even had a conversation with this person). This definitely classifies as stalking.

Geek Squad on Steroids

Cyberstalking has become an increasingly popular tool of harassment. Many victims find themselves being bombarded by e-mails or computer viruses or having their personal information spread all over the Internet by a cowardly harasser. Because of the vastness of the system, anonymity is quite easy to keep. Thanks to federal laws, task forces have popped up all over the country designed to combat this obnoxious and threatening behavior. For more information on cyberstalking and Internet safety, read Chapter 6, "Facebook = Open Book."

Me, Myself, and I

There also is a strange phenomenon of people who stalk themselves. This usually is a person who is trying to win back an ex-lover by pretending she is in danger, or someone who is extremely insecure and is falsely claiming she is being stalked to gain attention. Either way, a secure Safety Chick will not engage in this kind of behavior.

Review these examples of stalking carefully. If you or someone you know is a recipient of this kind of unwanted attention, there are several things to do to protect yourself.

Remember: THE KEY TO STAYING ALIVE AS A STALKING VICTIM IS TO STAY ONE STEP AHEAD OF YOUR STALKER.

Enough Is Enough—What to Do If You Are Being Stalked

1. Make Your Feelings Known.

The first moment your intuition tells you that the person's behavior is inappropriate, you should tell the stalker loud and clear, "I WANT NO FURTHER
CONTACT WITH YOU OF ANY KIND." Even if he does not comply, you can tell
the police that you have made your feelings clear to the stalker. Now his
behavior can be considered harassment.

2. Avoid Any Further Contact with the Stalker.

Sometimes this can be quite difficult. It might mean you have to shop somewhere
else, find new restaurants, even change your address. Many victims believe that they
should not have to turn their lives upside down because of a stalker. I wholeheartedly
agree, but until they can put all stalkers on an iceberg somewhere in the middle
of the Antarctic, your safety is more important than where you buy your groceries.
This also means never, *ever* communicate with a stalker in person, on the phone, or by
e-mail or snail mail. Any contact (even if you're screaming a stream of obscenities) can
be interpreted by the stalker as a sign of encouragement.

3. Document All Incidents.

Get a journal and write down the time, date, and description of every incident.
Whether it's a phone call or a sighting of the suspect parked in front of your home,
make a note of it. Even if you don't think it's important, the police will. In order
to charge a suspect with the crime of stalking, you need to show a laundry list of
harassing behavior. Every little bit helps. (See "The Safety Chick Stalking Incident
Log," page 204, for a form you can photocopy or tear out to use for documenting
stalking incidents.)

4. Notify the Police.

If the stalker persists after you have made it clear that you want no further
contact, notify the police. It is best to visit the campus police station and sit down
with an officer to make the report, rather than having a police officer and patrol
car come to your dorm (which can be conspicuous if you want to keep your case
private). Be clear and calm. Bring all evidence and documentation with you. The
police are there to help you, but you are the one who needs to facilitate your
own case. You need to work with the police in getting the stalker to stop the
threatening behavior. As I said earlier, we have come a long way legally since the

crime of stalking was given a name. While there are laws in every state, some police departments remain relatively mystified by the behavior. That's why it is so important for you to be a reliable and organized "client." If you still are not getting a good response from your local police, contact one of the victims' rights organizations listed on page 195.

5. Save All Evidence.

This means that ugly teddy bear that he left on your doorstep, the dead flowers he left on your desk, even the stupid Post-It note he left on your car. Make sure you save any telephone messages on your answering machine or voice mail as well. All of this is extremely helpful to the police and aids in the prosecution of the stalker.

6. Keep a Camera and/or Video Camera with You.

Snap his picture (using your cell phone is easiest) or videotape his antics on film. That's right, be your own detective. Remember, it's your word against his. The more concrete evidence, the better. This DOES NOT mean that you should put yourself in danger just to get the shot. Use your common sense.

7. Keep an Emergency Contact List.

Make sure you have an easily accessible list of names and numbers that could be critical in your time of need. For example: 911 (of course), the name of the police officer or detective who has been assigned to your case, your attorney or prosecutor, and any neighbors or family who can assist you.

8. Notify Family, Friends, Neighbors, and Coworkers That You Are Being Stalked.

For a lot of victims, this can be uncomfortable or embarrassing. I assure you, your personal well-being should outweigh any awkwardness. If you have a picture of your stalker, make copies for your trusted friends, family, neighbors, and roommates. If you know the suspect's name, vehicle description, and/or work and home addresses, distribute that information as well. Your neighbors can be your eyes and ears when you are not home, your roommates can ward off any unexpected visits from the stalker, and your family can be an essential support group for you in an incredibly stressful and emotional time.

9. Obtain a Restraining Order.

This is a legal document from the court that restricts the stalker from contacting you or coming near you in any way. Violators are subject to arrest. This is the first step in getting your tormentor prosecuted for the crime of stalking. But a restraining order is not always the answer. Sometimes (mostly in cases of domestic violence) this can be a catalyst to the stalker. Even a simple piece of paper restricting the stalker from getting near his victim can set off violent retaliation. In these cases, an alternate course of action should be taken. Filing a restraining order is something that should be discussed with the police officer or detective that has been assigned to your case. Bottom line: proceed with caution.

10. Believe in Yourself.

Being stalked is traumatic. Many victims feel that they have done something to make the stalker behave this way. Remember: IT IS NOT YOUR FAULT! Everyone in this world is responsible for their own actions. The prototypical stalker is emotionally weak and disturbed. You have done nothing to provoke this violating, destructive behavior. STAY STRONG!

Going Incognito—How to Keep Your Personal Information Private

I hope that none of you will ever have to go through being stalked. But even if this sad and frightening phenomenon has not touched your life, or even if it feels like a remote concept, every person should take certain security measures to keep personal information private so that stalkers and other criminals cannot access it. It took me several years to get all of this sorted out, and a lot of this information I learned through trial and error. I am sharing it with you here in as clear and helpful language as I can so you can use it readily and trial free.

Phone

- **Always request an unlisted phone number.** That way, *you* decide who has your number. It also cuts down on all those obnoxious telemarketers.
- **Never give your full name when signing up for service.** Just give your initial and last name, or—if possible—a different name completely. For example: T. Bono or T-Bone Enterprises.
- **Avoid giving out your home number to anyone except friends and family.** If you are having your car serviced or need to give a number to a store clerk, always provide a cell phone or work number. You never can be sure what these people will do with your number. Often they enter you in their database. The next thing you know, your private number is on every telemarketing list in

town. Now there is a much greater possibility of personal information falling into the wrong hands.

- **Do not list your home number in a directory of any kind.** Always use your cell phone or work number if you want to be listed in a club or school directory. People still will be able to reach you. Remember, if they are your friends, they already have your number.

Mail

- **Get a P.O. box.** You can go to the nearest post office or private mail center such as Mail Boxes Etc. and sign up. The difference between the U.S. Post Office and a private mail center is that at the post office they assign you a P.O box number, and they do not accept UPS or FedEx packages. Private mail centers give you an actual address and *will* accept packages. This is a bit more expensive than the post office, but might be worth it if you get a lot of parcels in the mail. Only give out your home address to friends and family. This not only cuts down on junk mail, it gives you a P.O. box number or address to list on your checks, driver's license, and other forms that circulate through the public sector and can therefore fall into the wrong hands.

- **Never list your name on your mailbox.** This includes dorms, apartments, and condominiums. Anyone who comes to your home should know your room or apartment number. If they don't, they shouldn't be there.

Rebecca Schaeffer, the actress from the popular 1980s TV sitcom *My Sister Sam*, was killed by a stalker on the front steps of her apartment building. She had her name listed right on the intercom system outside the building. Robert Bardo, who is serving life in prison, simply buzzed her apartment, which summoned her downstairs and into his waiting bullet.

- **Keep a lock on your mailbox.** One of the easiest ways that a person can find out all of your personal information is to intercept a document sent to you. If you cannot get a P.O. box, this is another way to protect your mail.

Remember: *You are the ruler of your private information.* Don't be bullied by companies wanting to put you on a mailing list, or a store clerk demanding your home address. Nobody is entitled to that information unless YOU say so.

Consistency helps you stay incognito from unwanted pursuers. Only YOU decide who gets to know your own "Private Idaho."

Survive a Stalker: The Extra Safety Chick Rules of Battle

There is nothing more debilitating than living like a hunted animal. If you find yourself in this weakened state, get your power back! Take control. I am NOT suggesting that you turn into the Terminator and hunt your stalker down. What I AM suggesting is that you take steps to decrease the chance of falling victim to your stalker. Here are some extra Safety Chick tips for the heat of battle:

Keep Your Intuition Antennae Way, Way Up!

When you leave or return to your home, take the time to drive up and down the streets for about a four-block radius. Scan every parked car for the stalker's vehicle. *I cannot tell you how many times this saved me from walking into my stalker's trap. Several times I saw his car parked down the street. Instead of going home, I would drive straight to the police station and make a report.* If you see the car, DO NOT approach it. Drive straight to the police station for help.

Curb Appeal

Stand at the front of your dorm, the front of your sorority house, or the entryway to your apartment. Look across the street, down the block, or around the corner. Where could a car park or person stand and watch your comings and goings? Once you have determined these locations, always scan the area when exiting or entering your home to make sure the stalker is not watching you from one of those positions. Make sure there are no obstacles blocking the front of your house from the street. If the police are driving by, they must be able to see your front door clearly. This is not paranoid behavior. This is a Safety Chick getting in touch with her surroundings.

Don't Panic, Get a Button

If you have filed a police report and are a victim of a stalker, check with your local victims' services office. ADT Security Services (see page 192) provides patrons with a necklace-type panic button, free of charge. When pressed, it calls the local police department directly for immediate help.

Set a Trap

Again, check with your local victims' services office and immediately have a trap set on your phone. Most phone service providers offer a free service for victims of harassing phone calls or a stalker if you have filed a report with the police department. They will install a device on your phone that keeps a record of who called you and when, even if the number is unlisted. Check and see if this service is offered in your community.

Miss Confidentiality

Most states offer the Address Confidentiality Program (ACP) through their attorney general's office. If you are a victim of a stalker, domestic violence, or sexual assault, you can designate the attorney general's office as your legal agent for processing legal documents and receiving mail. In return, you will be assigned a substitute address. The address has no relation to your home, work, or school address. Check with your state attorney general's office for more information on the ACP.

Be Resourceful

The crime of stalking is one of the most devastating offenses a victim can experience. Since 1997, we have had in the United States an anti-stalking law in every state and a federal law that protects victims, as well. Law enforcement agencies all over the country have taken the Los Angeles Police Department's lead and created anti-stalking departments within their divisions. If you are a victim, there are several places you can go to for help. The first is your local police station. There are also wonderful victims' rights organizations that can give further assistance if you need it. See Resources, page 195, for more information.

As I write this chapter, I have to be honest and tell you that it brings back a lot of raw emotion from my stalking ordeal. It is with that surviving emotion that I am able to write this book with such strong conviction. I am extremely proud of the progress our judicial system has made in prosecuting these manipulative predators—although that's not to say that there isn't still room for improvement, such as stronger sentencing for offenders. In my mind, the most constructive thing about the creation of the anti-stalking laws is that they actually stop violence before it escalates. Implementing the proper procedures allows police to arrest a criminal before he or she does physical harm to the victim. This may be the first law that by definition can actually prevent a rape or murder from happening! My hat goes off to U.S. Congressman Ed Royce, who pioneered the legislation from the very beginning. On behalf of Safety Chicks everywhere, he is to be commended.

Safety Chick Checklist:

What to Do If You Are Being Stalked

☒ **CLARIFY** | Make it clear to the stalker that you want no further contact.

☒ **DOCUMENT ALL INCIDENTS IN A JOURNAL** | Include time, date, and description of event.

☒ **SAVE ALL EVIDENCE** | Phone messages, e-mails, letters, gifts, etc.

☒ **CONTACT THE POLICE** | Bring all evidence to the police station.

☒ **CANDID CAMERA** | Keep a camera and/or video camera on hand. Snap his picture or videotape his antics. DO NOT put yourself in danger to get the shot. Stay in your car or home when taking the picture and make sure the environment is safe before you videotape any damage that has been done.

☒ **MAKE AN EMERGENCY CONTACT LIST** | Include phone numbers of the local police station, the name and badge number of the officer assigned to your case, school contact numbers, and the name and number of your attorney or the prosecutor, as well as any child care contacts, if necessary. Make sure both you and your family have a copy.

AVOID ANY FURTHER CONTACT WITH THE STALKER | Do not communicate with your stalker in any way. Change your daily routine. Shop at a different grocery store; drive home a different way every day. If your situation is extremely dangerous, relocate. (Talk with police officials or victims' assistance organizations for help; see page 195.)

SEE PAGE 204 FOR THE SAFETY CHICK STALKING INCIDENT LOG.

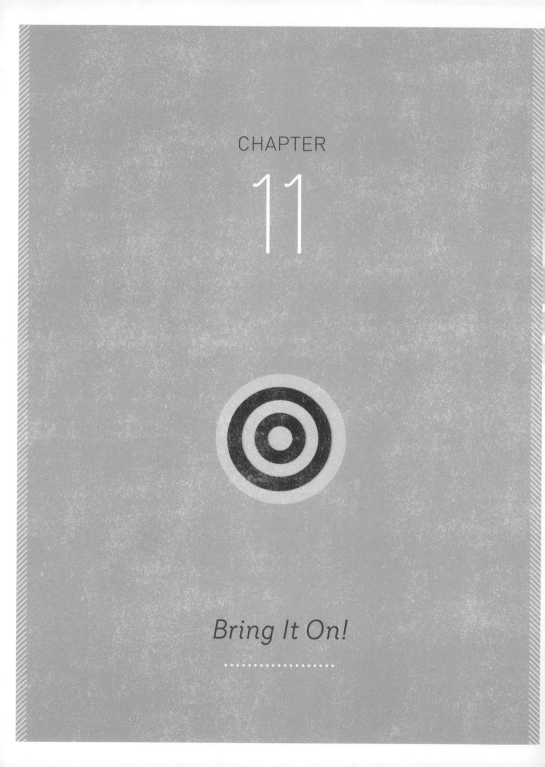

CHAPTER

11

Bring It On!

One evening in 2007, a student at the University of Arizona was leaving the library. She was walking to her car in the parking garage when suddenly she realized that someone was following her. She assessed the threat quickly because her awareness was heightened—there had been reports of a serial rapist on the loose. As she approached her car, she saw there was a person approximately three car lengths behind her. No one else was around. Luckily for her, her mom worked for the TASER company, and had given her an M26 TASER to carry. All she did was calmly pull out the gun-shaped TASER "stun gun," point it at the looming figure, and pull back the safety to expose the laser beam. A red dot was trained right on the guy's chest. Needless to say, he took off running. Shaken, the woman called the campus police and the predator was captured a few buildings down. He indeed was the rapist the police had been looking for. Thanks to the student's quick thinking—and Mom's TASER—she saved other potential rape victims from that criminal's attack.

Open a Can of Whoop-Ass: Methods of Self-Defense

I have two brothers. While we were growing up together, they used to terrorize me. They would pin me down and pretend to drip spit in my face, throw a bean bag chair on top of me and pretend to crush me—not exactly fun. But what I realized over the years is that unless they have brothers, most women have never wrestled or roughhoused like men have.

After watching my own three boys constantly wrestling and fighting with each other, I understand even more clearly why men have a distinct advantage over women when it comes to self-defense. Again, it isn't entirely their size or strength—it is probably largely also due to the fact that they are used to the feeling of getting punched, kicked, strangled, held down, and generally roughed up. (All in good fun, of course!) The idea of learning self-defense can be, for a lot of women, extremely intimidating. They are simply scared of the idea of physical violence, or feel that they are not strong enough to fend off an attacker. But, in the words of my friend Erin Weed, in her book *Girls Fight Back*, "the secret is this: Women do not fight men with strength. Women fight with strategy." The entire concept of the Safety Chick is that the odds of being a victim of a random act of violence are slim to none if you make smart personal-safety choices. BUT to truly live free and empowered, every woman should have the knowledge, confidence, and ability to protect herself in case it should ever come to that. I believe that every woman should take some type of self-defense class.

The story above shows that you don't necessarily have to get into hand-to-hand combat to thwart off an attack—the key is to find a deterrent that buys you time to get out of a dangerous situation, safely and unharmed. You have to be resourceful and use whatever technique you can. This chapter examines techniques of conflict resolution, as well as basic self-defense methods that can protect you in your time of need. Learning how to "open a can of whoop-ass," as Erin likes to put it, is essential to protecting yourself.

Remember that the key to staying alive in an attack is to not get there in the first place. Making smart personal-safety choices and practicing the routine of safety in numbers when out and about can alleviate the odds of ever having to use self-defense. But, in order to truly live free and empowered, you need to be ready to handle a threatening situation should it occur. Here are the most important things to know about basic self-defense.

"For to win one hundred victories in one hundred battles is not the ultimate skill. To subdue the enemy without fighting is the ultimate skill." **—Sun Tzu, 500 B.C.**

TIP #1 HOLD THAT THOUGHT—How to Get Out of a Potentially Violent Situation Before It's Too Late

As you probably guessed, the most important tool to use when assessing a threatening situation is your intuition (see Chapter 1). If you are walking down a sidewalk, use the reflection of a storefront window to track a potential attacker. If you are in a car, make a turn and then another to see if someone is following you. Using your intuition allows you to avert a potentially threatening situation. First and foremost, the key is to AVOID a potentially violent setting.

If you do find yourself face to face with a predator, there are several things you can do to dodge danger and, ultimately, save your life. The first thing is to understand who you are dealing with.

Matt Thomas is the creator of the highly acclaimed self-defense program, Model Mugging. Matt combines psychological empowerment with simple but effective defense moves. Model Mugging is the most efficient self-defense philosophy that I know, mainly because women finally get a chance to hit, punch, and kick full force. The "muggers" wear padded helmets and suits and do not hold back in their strength when attempting to attack. I believe this is invaluable practice for women. Getting to feel what it is actually like to be in a fight with a man is essential to knowing how to fend off an attacker.

Matt has a gift for turning an extremely physical and emotional process into common sense and empowerment. He has written a book called *Defend Yourself! Every Woman's Guide to Safeguarding Her Life.* I love this excerpt, which provides a great example of how wisdom can overcome fear:

Cowards in the Dark

An imaginary enemy is often more frightening than an actual one. When we are children, our greatest fears are often of monsters. As we get older, we may encounter children sometimes bigger than we are, who are bullies. Looking back with adult eyes, we know those monsters were not real and that the bullies were themselves afraid and insecure and, in most cases would have been cowards had we stood up to them.

The average rapist is not a huge monster but instead averages five feet eight inches tall and weighs one hundred and fifty pounds.

The average rapist is not a brave and fearless conqueror. He's a coward. All rapists are cowards! Research shows that in half of all rape attempts, any resistance from the woman causes the rapist to run away. The completion rate of rape against a single, unarmed woman is 33 percent. By contrast, the completion rate against a woman armed with a club, knife, or firearm is only 3 percent.

Men who attack women are, like people who make obscene phone calls, cowards in the dark, relying upon your fear. If you don't allow a man the power of intimidation, he may very likely run away to find a more cooperative victim.

Cowards, of course, can do great harm. But your fear of them is only useful if it propels you into meaningful action, and your best chance for that is if you respect the threat but also recognize your ability to stand up to it.

Men who commit violent offenses against women are nothing more than animals. Therefore, you need to understand how an animal thinks and behaves. Matt believes that in order to fully learn how to protect yourself against an attacker you must understand that the root of all attacks is based on the Prey vs. Predator mentality. What does a tiger do when his prey runs from him? He runs after the victim at full speed. The same is true for an attacker. If you turn and run, he will run you down. So, unless you are an Olympic sprinter or you have a clear shot to safety, you need to learn how to turn and face your predator with clarity and confidence.

Stop, Look, Assess

Whenever you are approached in a manner that you perceive as threatening, scan the area to assess the danger. There is always the possibility that your attacker is not alone. When you are in an adrenaline state, you can get a form of tunnel vision and might not see another attacker until it is too late. It is imperative that you use your peripheral vision as you take your stand. Force yourself to turn your head left and right to see exactly who you are dealing with.

The "Freeze Walk" Stance

Self-defense begins with a fighting stance—one that is designed to potentially defuse the situation without physical force and, at the same time, enables you to explode into decisive action. According to Matt, it is called the "freeze walk" because that is exactly how you learn it. You are walking. Suddenly your heart pounds, you've heard a sound (your *intuition* kicks in). Someone calls you or someone is coming toward you. You feel that you are in danger. Stop and face the direction of the danger. Again, do not run unless you know where you're running to and have absolute confidence that you can escape.

Wax On, Wax Off

This is a good visual for your arm movement. Quickly bend your elbows in and swing your forearms and hands in front of your face in a half circle. As you execute this move, say "No!" in a low, serious growl. Done right, this move can appear to the attacker that you are not offering a challenge but that you are acknowledging and respecting his potential power. It tells him that he has nothing to prove.

You aren't communicating *"Back off, creep!"* but rather, "Stop, you are making me uncomfortable and invading my space." You have now, rather than staging a confrontation that could escalate the danger, set a boundary that tells your attacker not to approach.

The two advantages of the "freeze walk" stance from a self-defense perspective are:

1. You have the opportunity to take the attacker by surprise because you have given him no sign of resistance.
2. Because he anticipates no fight, he will probably try to grab you, therefore making it easier for you to defend yourself.

Put on a Show—The Threat Display

The next step is to show your "threat display." Think of an alley cat when it is approached by an unfamiliar feline: back arched and tail fluffed, usually making a growl or sound of warning. Body language is everything. You must speak to your attacker's "inner core," which is animalistic. You do not want to appear threatening, but you also don't want to appear weak. Be calm and firm and in control.

Two Little Letters; Big, Big Word

There are many reasons as to how and why saying the word "no" can be the difference between life and death.

1. Forcefully saying "NO!" in a low-guttural voice startles your attacker and throws him off guard.
2. Using a loud threatening growl instead of a helpless whimper or scream sends a message to your predator (think of animals when they fight; the one that growls wins, the one that whimpers loses).
3. Exhaling "NO!" replaces the natural inhale of fear with the exhale breath of anger.
4. The word "NO!" said in a stern manner is a command to stop behavior that all mothers direct at their children. This might trigger the criminal's subconscious and throw him off.
5. A loud growl attracts attention, a loud scream frightens people. Onlookers have a tendency to stop to watch a fight; therefore, someone might stop to help. If you scream, people might be frightened and run away.

In addition to a threat display and establishing boundaries, you also need to give the attacker an option to de-escalate. This is a statement that should be made after you have said "No."

Talk 'Em Down

Using a phrase like, "Leave me alone, I don't want any trouble" in a commanding growl gives the assailant a chance to back off. Do not say, "I'm going to kick your ass!" No matter how tempted you might be, these words excite an attacker, and could be his invitation to fight.

Sticks and Stones

One of the easiest and most intimidating weapons an attacker can use is words. Vile, scary words said in an abusive and threatening way are terrifying, if you allow them to be. So do not be intimidated by his words. Focus instead on his actions. Pump yourself up by saying to yourself, "Come on, buddy, is that the best you can do?" or "Yeah, well, your Mama didn't raise you right." Don't let his words break your concentration.

No Fisticuffs

Make sure that your hands are not making a fist; this sends a signal to the predator to use fists back. Hands in front of your face with fingers spread allows you to be in the "ready" position without signaling to your attacker that you are set to punch.

According to Matt Thomas, 750 women who took the Model Mugging course reported attempted attacks against them by predators after taking the class. Of those, 550 were able to thwart their potential attackers just by using the voice and stance of a threat display. Remember, a predator is nothing more than an animal. Anything that you can do to shake up his pattern gives you a chance to escape and avert an attack.

ALL TOGETHER NOW

These moves should be performed all together in a fluid motion.

1. Stop, turn, and assess the situation. Turn your head to the left and right to properly scan the area.
2. Get into a firm stance: Feet shoulder-width apart, one foot slightly in front of the other, hips square.
3. As you forcefully say the word "No," arms smoothly swing up in front of your face, fingers spread, hands wave slightly, elbows are as close together as you can get them.
4. Follow up with, "Leave me alone, I don't want any trouble."

You have set the stage for what happens next. It is now up to your attacker to lead you into your next move.

If you have made every move you know to get out of a threatening situation and you are still in danger, you must now Open Your Can of Whoop-Ass. In the next section, I will teach you three moves that you can use in various combinations to defend yourself effectively. But first I want you to understand how to pick your battleground and utilize your surroundings. If you are in front of a plate glass window, move away. If you are on stairs, move up or down. The key is to remove yourself from an area that your attacker could use against you, and to take control.

Obstacle Course

If a predator is making his way toward you, put a physical obstacle between you and him. For example, get on the other side of a parked car, lamp post, magazine rack—anything that makes him work to get to you. This throws him off balance. If he has to come between two parked cars, take that opportunity to step to the side of one of the cars, wait for him to step between the two. And then let him have it. If you can jump behind a thorny bush or hedge, go for it. Predators don't like to work too hard for their prey. Make it tough; wear him down. If you are on a sidewalk, make him step off the curb and hit him when he's mid-step. Stairs are tricky because you don't want to be thrown down them. If you have a chance to make him step up or step down, however, do it. Remember, getting your attacker off balance is the key. Use your surroundings to your advantage.

When in Doubt, Improvise

Improvised weapons are a great addition to your self-defense moves. They can be found just about anywhere and are quite effective against a predator. Matt has classified these into three categories: projectile weapons, club weapons, and cutting weapons.

Projectile weapons are things that can be thrown into your assailant's eyes that can temporarily blind him or cause him to lift his head, enabling you to do a heel palm strike (see page 179) to the nose. Common things are sand, dirt, coins, or hot coffee. (Remember the woman who sued McDonald's because she spilled coffee on her lap as she was driving away? That stuff burns!)

Club weapons are objects that you can use to jab or hit your attacker. Aim for the head; usually your attacker will grab the object. Take that opportunity to go for his privates, one of the most vulnerable areas for men. Common objects can be a purse, umbrella (club and jab), briefcase, or backpack. Remember: Let go if he grabs the object. You do not want to be pulled off balance; the goal is to cause a distraction so you can remove yourself from harm's way. If your object has a sharp end like an umbrella or pen, jab at the eye or neck.

Cutting weapons are implements such as knives, nail files, broken glass, or bottles. The best place to use these weapons on your attacker is the eyes, face, or neck. However, Matt does not recommend using these in hopes of stopping the attack cold. Knife wounds rarely incapacitate a person. In fact, many people don't even realize they've been stabbed for minutes after an attack.

Improvised weapons are to be used against your attacker as a distraction to enable you to make your move. Any of these will be a deterrent to the predator, but probably not a disabler. You must be ready to use your self-defense moves to do the rest.

A model in New York once fended off an attacker by beating him about the face and head with the heel of her Ferragamo pumps and her Chanel purse.

If someone is wielding a knife or sharp object at you, wrap a jacket or sweater around your hand and forearm to fend off the attack. Swing your arm in a figure-eight motion.

Target Practice

Before you learn how to hit, you need to know where to hit. Chances are, your attacker will be bigger and stronger than you. To compensate for that, you must hit him where he is most vulnerable. According to Matt, there are two places: the groin and the nose.

Hit Below the Belt

No matter how big and strong a man is, he can be incapacitated by a forceful blow to the genitals. Use the front of your thigh, not your knee. Do not aim for the front of the body. Instead, thrust your thigh up and under the groin. The idea is to crush the testicles up into their pelvic bone. *(Ouch!)*

Be Nosey

The other highly vulnerable part of a man's body is the nose. Take the butt of your hand and lightly tap your nose—see how much it hurts? Just a little bonk can cause your eyes to water or shut. A forceful strike to the nose can cause blurred vision, bleeding, dizziness, a broken bone, even unconsciousness. Even if you miss the nose, a blow to the face or head will do some damage.

The One-Two Punch

There are two target areas—focus on them and strike whichever is most accessible.

Because the two target points are at different parts of his body, he cannot defend both areas at once. So, the idea is not to knock him out with one punch, but rather, keep the pummeling going until he is unconscious or gets the hell away from you.

If he covers his groin, go for the nose; when he guards his face, go for his testicles. If he's grabbing for your arms, you've still got your legs. If he grabs your legs, you've still got your arms. You become a lean, mean fighting machine before he knows what hit him.

How to Rumble in the Jungle

Now that you know why to hit, who to hit, and where to hit, you need to know HOW to hit. From the threat-display stance (one foot slightly in front of the other, hips square), your first defensive strike is at the upper target: the nose. Matt calls this potentially powerful punch the "heel-palm strike." He teaches this punch for several reasons; primarily because it is very easy to learn (mastering the correct way of performing a fist-punch so as not to break the knuckle or wrist can take years) and also because the positioning of the heel-palm strike allows you to keep your hands up in a protective position. So, if you miss the blow, you can still protect yourself against your attacker.

Palm Power

If you put enough power behind the base of your palm, you can break any man's nose. From your threat-display stance, a heel-palm strike is an easy and natural move. If your right foot is back, lead with your right palm. If your left foot is back, lead with your left palm. The move is sudden and explosive. The striking arm extends while the same hip thrusts (and slightly twists) forward; most of the power comes from below the waist. All momentum and power should be focused on the attacker's nose. Don't forget to yell "NO!" with every strike. Your other hand stays up, elbow bent, protecting your face.

Mastering the Move

Do not fully extend the arm during the move—it can give you a hyperextended elbow (bad for your tennis game). Jab forward until the elbow is only slightly bent, then pull back to the protective hands-up position. Keeping the elbows in, parallel with your shoulders, allows you to deliver a powerful offensive strike. In addition, when thrusting your palm forward, you can deflect an oncoming inside jab to your face. When bringing your arm back to the guard position, you can deflect an outside jab to the side of your head. (Now you're movin'.)

"Keep in mind that our number one objective is not to cause pain to an attacker, but to cause disability." **—Erin Weed, Girls Fight Back**

Push 'em Back, Push 'em Back, Waaay Back

Part of the objective of this move is to knock your attacker backward, away from you. When you strike his nose, imagine your hand driving into his skull. Matt thinks a good way to practice the heel-palm strike is to kneel on a mat or firm mattress and alternate the right and left strike in repetitions of three. Yell "No" with each strike (be sure to tell family members that you are practicing your moves). Concentrate on the heel of the palm striking the surface with force. Shake your body out after every repetition.

My, What Lovely Thighs You Have

The heel-palm strike will draw the attacker's attention to his head, and may cause him to bleed, and get teary-eyed and dizzy. In any case, he will have exposed his other target area for you to pummel. Your next move is the "thigh-to-groin move." Use the thigh of the leg that is back and drive it forward, under his groin with the portion of the thigh bone closest to your knee. Shout "No," then step forward. Make sure to keep your hands up, because this move will put you right next to your attacker to drive your thigh up, under, and through. Like the heel-palm strike, this move is sudden and explosive.

Perfecting the Move

Done correctly, the thigh-to-groin move can lift your assailant off the ground, crushing the testicles to the pelvic bone. Quite a problem if your attacker is trying to commit sexual assault. Even if you miss the groin, a strike to the thigh, hip, or abdomen creates pain and/or distraction, which will cause him to expose his other target: the nose and head. Practice the thigh-to-groin move in slow motion, three times with each leg.

Stay A"Head" of the Game

If the attacker isn't lying on his back or side by now, then he will (as any man will tell you) bend forward, holding his groin, his head unguarded. Keep moving forward and drive the other thigh into his head and shout, "No!" There isn't a specific target on the head; anywhere is fine—you don't want to rely on fine motor skills when you are in an adrenaline state. Aim for the center of the head, but a solid blow to any part of the head can knock him out. As with the thigh-to-groin move, the thigh-to-head is a thrust forward with the entire body that should drive your thigh up at his head. (Think of driving a football through the uprights for an extra point with your thigh.)

Practice the thigh-to-groin move followed by the thigh-to-head move. (It's like a high step with one leg and then a high step with the other.) Then practice all three moves together: Heel-palm strike to the nose/high step forward with same side leg/thigh-to-groin move/high step forward with other leg/thigh-to-head move. With each move, yell the word, "No!"

These moves need to become second nature, so you must practice the entire sequence together. Practicing in front of a mirror helps; doing so with girlfriends is even better!

Practice in sequences of three and rest before doing another three. Keep in mind that these moves are a response to a very specific kind of attack—frontal and standing by an unarmed assailant. However, the "freeze walk" stance and the high/low target area combination moves provide the basis for all other defense moves.

Not an Exact Science

Remember, every situation is different. There is no way to prepare for what exactly might happen if you are ever approached by an attacker. The key is to become extremely comfortable with the three moves, and just keep repeating them on your assailant until he retreats or falls to the ground.

Get a Little Closer

As uncomfortable as this may sound, the closer you are to your assailant, the better. In order to perform these moves effectively, you must get as close to the attacker as possible. The urge will be to push away, but doing so allows the attacker to get the advantage. Staying in close and using your heel-palm strike to the nose and thigh to the groin and head gives you a fighting chance.

We All (Might) Fall Down

If your attacker is able to push you to the ground or you accidentally fall, be ready. Practice falling backward from the standing position, using a gymnastics type mat or mattress. With your hands in the ready position, cross one foot in back of the other, bend your knees, and gently fall down. Be sure to keep your hands up, and let your legs and rear end absorb the fall. Use your stomach muscles to keep you upright and quickly roll onto your side. Many a wrist has been broken by putting an arm out to absorb a fall. Falling hurts, but falling the right way allows you to continue defending yourself without incurring serious injury.

I Get a Kick Out of You

Once you hit the ground, roll to your side. If you are on your right side, get up on your right forearm (not your elbow), left hand touching the ground for balance. Immediately start kicking with the top leg. Slightly bend the bottom leg and use the top leg as you would your arm. Think of the heel-palm strike, but with the heel and bottom of your foot. Aim for the head and groin. If your attacker bends over to try to attack, kick his head. As he falls back from the kick, aim for the groin. Use your arms and butt to pivot around as your attacker moves. A good visual is that your arms and butt and bottom leg are on a lazy Susan and your top leg is a powerful piston pumping into your chest and out, forcefully kicking your target points. Done right, when performing the kick, your chest will almost be touching the ground as you rotate your hips forward and propel your flexed foot and leg toward the target. This is called the "side thrust kick." (You may find it easier to think of it as a side/back kick.)

Sometimes having a power bootie really pays off. All of your kicking power is derived from the gluteus maximus muscle. Focus and tap into that large muscle group. Bring the knee into your chest and drive your foot out with your "bootylicious" (the phrase made immortal by songstress chicks Destiny's Child) strength. Get into position and practice this kick in slow motion. Focus on your target, looking over your shoulder. In your mind, aim for the head and groin areas. Practice three times on each leg. Make sure to follow through with the leg. Always practice the moves with complete follow-through. Stopping short of your target or drawing back your leg before full extension is a bad habit to get into. Remember: When you are in an adrenaline state, you do what you have practiced. Pulling back before you hit your target isn't going to do you much good in the heat of battle.

Like Riding a Bike

If you end up on the ground and can't get to the side, use a "front thrust kick." To get the power for this kick, you must be up on your forearms and rear end. Think of peddling a bicycle in the air. It is a one-two combination. Aim for the head and groin; one foot high, one foot low. (Don't forget to yell, "No" with every kick.) This kick doesn't have as much power as the side thrust kick, but it does have the advantage of fast repetitions and easier accuracy. Remember: He can't protect both areas at the same time, so look for the target opening and keep going for it. Picture yourself playing the game at the carnival where you smack the gopher with a wooden mallet when he pops out of his hole. The mallets are your powerful legs, and the holes are the unprotected target areas of your gopher—I mean, assailant.

Give 'em the Ax, the Ax, the Ax

(That title is for all of my Stanford friends.) The last effective kick is called the "ax kick." This kick should be used when your attacker is down but not unconscious, or if he is getting up to try to attack you again. The move is simple and is done in the same position as the side thrust kick. Bring your top knee in toward your chest, but this time bring your leg up and swing your flexed foot down on his head or groin like an ax. The leg should remain slightly bent through the whole kick. Practice this three times on each side on your bed or mat, again yelling "No!" with each repetition.

It's Combo Time

Now, practice falling. Get used to the feeling of using your legs and rear end rather your arms to break your fall. Quickly roll to the side and practice your side thrust kicks, transition right into the front kicks, and finish with the ax kick. Repeat three times on each side. To really get comfortable, practice various combinations in any order. Remember: There is no exact science to self-defense. The more ways you practice, the more situations you're prepared for.

Rising from the Ashes

Finally, your attacker has stopped moving. He is either tired or unconscious, or faking it. Proceed with caution. Carefully swing your legs around and stand up. Be aware of your surroundings. Walk toward your attacker with your hands in the ready position. Step above his head, but out of his reach and yell, "No." Quickly assess your situation. Is he getting up? Is someone else coming toward you? Are they friend or foe? If your attacker is getting up, begin using the defense moves again. If he is unconscious, find someone to call 911 for you. Take a deep breath; try to calm down and realize that your mind and body just went through an extremely emotional and powerful event. Focus on the positive: You were incredibly strong you had tremendous courage and you used your inner wisdom— definitely a Self-Defense Safety Chick.

There are many more moves and defense scenarios in the Model Mugging training. Because this is not solely a self-defense book, I am not able to cover them all. The moves that I have covered should give you a really good foundation. But, I recommend taking a self-defense class like Model Mugging to train appropriately. For more information on Model Mugging, look to the Resources section at the end of the book (page 196).

Take That, Hot Shot! The Differences in Pepper Sprays, Pepper Foams, and Other Self-Defense Aerosols

Before you choose to carry a pepper spray or foam, realize that there are certain conditions when these products might not be the right choice. For example, if you are in an enclosed area, spraying your attacker with pepper spray can also mean that you are spraying yourself. If you are using an aerosol, rain or wind can affect where the spray ends up. However, defense sprays are still among the easiest and most effective protection products you can use.

Defense Spray 101

Self-defense sprays are made up of irritating and inflammatory agents. They can include combinations of tear gas, hot cayenne peppers, and ultraviolet dye. The spray can reach anywhere from 8 to 20 feet, depending on the model, and can incapacitate an assailant for anywhere from 20 to 90 minutes.

Shed a Tear

While it is classified separately from tear gas, pepper spray works like one. It's an irritant. Sprayed in an assailant's face, it can cause extreme pain. It can cause the eyes to water and make breathing difficult. The pain also can cause a feeling of panic. But if your assailant is on alcohol or drugs of any kind, he might not feel the pain and be able to keep functioning.

Spray or Foam

There are pepper sprays and pepper foams. The difference between them is simple: One shoots like a spray of kitchen cleaner and the other shoots like a stream of foam. The pepper spray is easy because it covers a larger area, so if you miss the eyes but spray around the head or face, the aerosol will still do its job. The drawback is lack of effectiveness in wind, rain, or an enclosed area. Then the foam is a better choice, as long as you shoot it directly into the attacker's face.

A Little Spitfire Does the Trick

Ultimately, pepper sprays can be ineffective when dealing with an attacker. Most canisters only spray when held straight up vertically and directly in your attacker's face, so the odds of a successful hit if you are attacked from behind or in a struggle are low. That is why Walter Cardwell, president and founder of Spitfire, came up with this great solution. The Spitfire is a bullet-shaped container that fits in the palm of your hand. You can keep it on your keychain ready to use when you are getting from point A to point B. The reason Spitfire works so well is that it can be shot from any angle—horizontal, vertical, whatever. It has a special valve that can shoot eight shots from eight feet in half-second bursts. The small device allows you to shoot from the hip or over your shoulder if you are attacked from behind, thus catching your attacker by surprise. I have shot it; it definitely works well. Another plus is that the bullet-shaped container can be used as a weapon on the pressure points of your attacker. Visit their Web site to learn about the Spitfire and how to use it (see Resources, page 196). The company also offers replaceable cartridges that easily pop into the container once yours is empty.

Take-Down Time

Several factors can determine how fast your attacker will be affected by a self-defense spray. Drugs or alcohol in the recipient's system can slow down the impact. Most normal take-down times are within seconds. In some instances, however, it can take a bit longer, so be prepared. Make sure you are a safe distance away from the attacker before you spray, so that you are not contaminated, as well.

Legal Issues

Defense sprays carry restrictions in some states. For example, in New York you can only purchase these sprays through a licensed firearms dealer or pharmacist. In Massachusetts, you must purchase defense sprays through licensed firearms dealers. In Michigan, you can carry no stronger than a 2 percent concentrate of pepper spray. CS (Containment Spray) is the only type of tear gas accepted and can be no larger than 35 grams per can. No combination sprays are allowed (meaning a combination of tear gas and pepper spray). In Wisconsin, no tear gas of any kind is allowed. You can only carry pepper spray and the container can have no stronger than a 10 percent concentrate in it. It must be between 15 and 60 grams in size and must have a safety-lock feature. The best thing to do to ensure your legal safety is to check with your local police department on defense spray policies. It is up to you to find out exactly where and when it is legal to carry and use pepper or any other type of spray.

Effects of Pepper Spray

During a TV show I did for Fox, they actually shot a guy with pepper spray right in the face. Now, granted, he was prepared to be sprayed—his body was ready for it and a paramedic was standing by. The effects of the pepper were excessive: tearing and burning of the eyes, coughing, and general discomfort. He said that he could still function, but not as forcefully and deliberately as before the spray. After the show, he flushed his eyes for several minutes with water and took in a little oxygen. When he left the set several minutes later, he was still not back to normal.

I want to reiterate that defense sprays are to be used as a deterrent—a product that allows you to disable your attacker long enough to get away from him. Because of the ease of use, this is the most popular form of defense product sold.

Don't TASE Me, Sis!: How and Why to Use a Civilian TASER C2

Stun guns, now most commonly known by their brand name TASER, offer more debilitating options when thinking about buying a personal-safety device. I believe that, much like a first-aid kit, your personal-safety kit should include many items. Pepper spray can protect you in certain situations; for example, if someone tries to grab you or your purse, a squirt of pepper spray in his eyes can temporarily blind him, buying yourself the opportunity to get out of harm's way. My Date Rape Coaster (available at www.thesafetychick.com) can protect you in others, like at a bar, or in social situations where you fear your drink has been tampered with. A TASER can protect you in others, such as if someone breaks into your home or you are being threatened on the street. Learning about all the self-defense products available makes you a more informed and empowered Safety Chick.

The Man Behind the TASER

I have been a fan of TASER for years, way before they came out with the civilian TASER (the old model looked like a gun and was used mostly by police officers) . . . heck, even back when they tried to market the not-so-successful "Auto TASER" (it was like a LoJack with a zap). I had the wonderful opportunity to meet Rick Smith, the cofounder of TASER, a few years ago at a law enforcement conference. I was so excited to meet him that I rambled on and on about how much I like the device and how I thought all women should own a TASER. His eyes lit up and he said, "Stay right there, I will be right back." He returned a few moments later with a small, sleek device that looked a little bigger than a cell phone—to my delight, it was a sparkly pink civilian TASER! I said it was great, but recommended that he make them in all kinds of colors that would appeal to women, even leopard print. Well, we struck up a very special friendship that day, and I ended up being a part of the company's infomercial, and even helped Rick, his brother Tom, and their awesome team launch the leopard print pattern (no longer available) C2 at the Consumer Electronics Show in Las Vegas.

It is a shame how the media has misinformed and poorly portrayed the TASER as a lethal weapon—the science just does not back up that theory. The whole reason Rick founded the company was because two of his high school friends were shot and killed in a senseless road rage incident. His passion and mission were to create a non-lethal personal-protection device, and that's what led to the TASER technology. (For more information on the science behind the product, visit www.taser.com.)

The C2

I really do not want this to sound like an infomercial for TASER—but, simply, one of the most effective uses for the device is if you are home and a criminal breaks in. The C2 is one of the best things you can have to protect yourself, your friends, and loved ones. Again (for the last time), personal safety is just that, personal. YOU decide what works best for you. The personal-safety products I am highlighting in this chapter are just suggestions, but ones that I have had experience using and believe in. The reason a TASER C2 is such a great choice is because it is easy to use, easy to shoot, and can hit your assailant from 15 feet away—thus removing the hand-to-hand combat issue I have talked about previously. It buys you time to get out of the house or situation you are in. When loaded with a cartridge, a simple press of a button shoots out two wires with hooks on the end. It also has a laser that points a red dot on your target making it really easy to aim. It shoots much like a New Year's Eve popper with confetti. The little dots of colored paper have serial numbers on them that are registered to the owner of the TASER—much like ballistics of a bullet shot from a gun, only much easier to track down. The wires reach 15 feet and can attach through 2 inches of clothing.

How the C2 Works

The wires conduct energy that affects the sensory and motor functions of the nervous system. Basically, it scrambles the sensory and motor signals to the brain, rendering the person incapacitated. I know this because I was shot by a TASER myself. No, not because I was climbing onstage at an Earth, Wind, and Fire concert, but because I was training to be a law enforcement instructor for TASER. I figured if I was going to talk about it to the national media, I better know of what I spoke. So, I took the "five second ride" (that's cop speak for getting shot by a TASER). All I can say is that I could not move once the prongs hit me, but when it stopped, I was perfectly fine and able to get up like nothing had happened (except for the holes in my T-shirt from the hooks).

Why the C2 Works

When you are in a life-threatening situation, you shake from nerves. The C2 shoots quick and easy. Just pointing the laser at the target and pressing the button allows you to hit your mark. If an attacker comes into your home or approaches you on the street, you don't have to wait until he is right in your face. You can be standing in your bedroom and if a predator enters your home, you can shoot from 15 feet away. If he comes toward you in a parking garage, you can drop him a few cars away. The point is, it keeps him away from you before you have to get into a hand-to-hand combat situation.

The TASER C2 renders your attacker incapacitated for fifteen seconds. You can either drop the TASER and run to safety, or opt to get the phone while you are holding the TASER, call 911, and press the button again to keep him on the ground until the police arrive. Remember: The best choice for you is to drop it, run, and get to safety.

If you decide to own and carry a TASER, it is crucial that you practice using it. It comes with an instructional DVD, but ultimately you need to get out in an open area with a target and a couple of cartridges and practice. And remember: You must be eighteen years old or older to own a TASER.

Don't worry about losing your TASER in the chaos of a confrontation: TASER's policy is, if you use the C2 for protection, all you have to do is send them the police report of the incident, and they will replace it free of charge.

TASER FYIs

If one of the prongs misses your attacker and he is still approaching, just touch the TASER to his body; it will complete the circuit and he will drop. The term is called a "drive stun."

When the cartridge is not in the TASER, it is a still a "stun gun." Just touch the device to the target's body and press the button—it will shock him and give you minutes in the aftermath to get away.

The best way to use the TASER is to shoot your target while standing a couple of feet away. The talons work best when they are about 16 inches apart to receive the best t-wave flow—meaning the best locations to get the best flow of current.

While the TASER will leave your attacker dazed and confused for several minutes, it has no aftereffects on muscles, nerves, or any other body function.

You're Stunning

Stun weapons generally are between the 7-and 14-watt range. They interrupt the body's signals to the nervous system, which makes a person unable to physically function (a very small percentage of people can have a high tolerance for electrical stimulation and can fight through it). Stun guns come in different voltages and different forms. The voltage does no permanent damage, but immobilizes the attacker for several minutes. Even if the attacker is touching you, the current will not pass to your body. The voltage delivers a pulse frequency that tells muscles to work at a rapid pace. This process converts blood sugar to lactic acid. If you have ever exercised too much one day and tried to get out of bed the next, you can identify with the feeling. That is a mild example, however. A 1-second, 600,000-volt charge can stop an attacker in his tracks, causing him to drop to the ground with intense muscle spasms, feeling dazed and confused for up to 15 minutes. A five-second charge can leave him feeling like he fell from a two-story building and landed on a bed of concrete. The downside is that you must be touching him to make the stun gun work—again, getting yourself into a hand-to-hand combat situation. Stunning him gives you an advantage, but you'd better act quickly to get out of harm's way.

Legal Guidelines

I have to emphasize again, it is up to you to check with your local law enforcement about restrictions or laws pertaining to owning a stun device. States where it is currently illegal to own stun devices are Hawaii, Massachusetts, Michigan, New Jersey, New York, Rhode Island, Wisconsin, and the District of Columbia. Even though a state might have no restrictions, cities within that state might. In Chicago, Baltimore, Philadelphia, and New York City, it is illegal to carry a stun device. Even states that allow stun devices have some sort of restrictions attached. For example, in Connecticut, you must have a written permit issued and signed by the mayor, chief of police, or other person of appropriate authority. That is why it is imperative that you check with authorities before you purchase any type of self-defense weapon.

Remember: The choice to carry or use self-defense or personal-safety products is up to you. You must act responsibly and fully understand the laws and any restrictions the device might carry and how to use the product effectively and efficiently. Practice with your device or product in a controlled environment, preferably with trained professionals on a regular basis. That is the Safety Chick way: Be prepared and ready to go should the situation call for defense.

Safety Chick Checklist:
Self-Defense Sequence

✖ **SCAN THE SITUATION** | Be aware of your surroundings.

✖ **FREEZE-WALK STANCE** | Threat display, establish boundaries, option to de-escalate.

✖ **HEEL-PALM STRIKE** | Heel of palm to his nose while shouting "No!"

✖ **THIGH-TO-GROIN MOVE** | Upper thigh of one leg thrusts up and under groin while shouting, "No!"

✖ **THIGH-TO-HEAD MOVE** | Second thigh thrusts into attacker's head while shouting, "No!"

✖ **ASSESS** | Make sure assailant is unconscious or incapacitated.

✖ **GET HELP** | Ask someone to call 911.

Resources—S.O.S.!

In this section, you will find all of the Web sites, agencies, and organizations for safety counsel and support that I have referred to throughout the chapters of this book (many thanks to all who helped me write such a comprehensive book), as well as others that might help you with more information. I have broken them down by chapter and subject. If you can't find what you are looking for, you can always contact me through my Web site www.safetychick.com for further assistance.

CHAPTER 2: Intro to Campus Safety

International Association of College Law Enforcement Administrators
www.iaclea.org | Provides helpful resources for public safety issues on all college or university campuses.

The Office of Victims Services in the Department of Justice
www.ojp.usdoj.gov/ovc/help/cc.htm | If you or someone you know has been a crime victim on campus and want to learn more about how to get help, go to the vast resources of this organization.

Safe Campuses Now
kathrynkeithsims@yahoo.com | The wonderful organization started by Dana Getzinger Foley at the University of Georgia has now been passed on to Kathryn (Keith) Sims, who has taken the Web site and created one of the most comprehensive safety resource sites for college students everywhere.

Security on Campus
www.securityoncampus.org | The national organization created by the parents of Jeanne Cleary in honor of their daughter. This is an incredible organization that is dedicated to keeping students safe from crime.

Safety Preparedness Index
www.rd.com | The *Reader's Digest* site offers a downloadable version of the index.

International Association of Chiefs of Police
www.iacp.org | IACP consists of over 20,000 operating chief executives of international, federal, state, and local agencies, and the organization has the most cutting-edge information relating to crime prevention.

The Center for Personal Protection and Safety (CPPS)
www.cppssite.com | This organization offers tons of travel safety tips. It is also the parent organization of the Safe Travel Institute (www.safe-travels.com) and National Hostage Survival Training Center.

University of Wisconsin Police Department
www.uwpd.wisc.edu/pmcscs.html | The UWPD has a great page on school shooting prevention.

CHAPTER 3: Welcome to My "Crib"

The College Board
www.collegeboard.com | A start-to-finish resource for being safe and successful at college.

Home Security
You can find home security products in most hardware stores. Window locks and portable alarm systems can also be found online. Two good sites are www.adt.com (for home security systems) and www.hometips.com (for easy how-to instructions on installation of window locks and other products).

Portable Security

www.computersecurity.com | Good resource for portable security locks and alarms for your computer. They have great products to keep your laptop and other products safe.

Rental Housing

www.residentassistant.com | This is an in-depth site that can help with any dorm or housing issues you might have. If you need more assistance or have other questions about apartment rentals, check out www.apartmentguide.com or www.move.com.

The Safety Chick Door Wedge alarm for your dorm, apartment, or hotel room makes your door hard to open from the outside and has a motion sensor with a 120-decibel alarm that will sound if someone attempts to open the door. This can be found on the products page at www.safetychick.com.

The U.S. Department of Housing and Urban Development

www.hud.gov | The helpful people at this organization will answer any questions or assist you with problems you might be having with landlords, roommates, etc.

CHAPTER 4: BFFs, Sisters, and All That Jazz

Anti-Hazing

www.stophazing.org | An organization dedicated to stopping hazing behavior on college campuses and general hazing/bullying everywhere.

www.hazingprevention.org | A great resource to learn more about hazing on college campuses and how to prevent it from happening.

Eating Disorders

www.eatingdisordersonline.com | This is a community-based site with members and blogging. It is the Internet's fastest growing eating-disorders community, and has the goal of bringing together people around the issue of eating disorders by providing concise, up-to-date information and a meeting place for those seeking pathways to recovery.

www.eating-disorder.com | A comprehensive site that can help you find a treatment center that is right for you, along with information and motivational stories of women who have overcome disorders.

www.nationaleatingdisorders.org | If you want to learn more about eating disorders, visit the excellent Web site of the National Eating Disorders Association.

www.somethingfishy.org | This site is part of the CRC Health Group, which is the nation's leading provider of treatment and educational programs for adults and youth who are struggling with behavioral issues, chemical dependency, eating disorders, obesity, pain management, or learning disabilities.

Empowerment

www.annbrashares.com | Ann Brashares, the author of *The Sisterhood of the Traveling Pants*, has a fabulous Web site along with a great list of books.

www.rosalindwiseman.com | Rosalind Wiseman, author of *Queen Bees & Wannabes*, has wonderful empowerment programs.

Sorority Information

www.thesororitylife.com | An excellent magazine and Web site about sorority life.

Stress Management

www.sleepfoundation.org | For information about how various factors affect sleep, and for aids on improving sleep.

www.stress.about.com | For more information on stress, its symptoms, and ways to cope.

CHAPTER 5: Watch It, Party Girl!

Alcohol

www.niaaa.nih.gov | Refer to the National Institute on Alcohol Abuse if you or someone you know has a problem with alcohol.

www.collegebingedrinking.net | This is one of the most comprehensive sites on binge drinking and alcoholism in young adults, and it is an incredible resource for dealing with addiction.

Advocacy
www.swhr.org | The Society for Women's Health Research (SWHR) is a national nonprofit organization based in Washington, DC, dedicated to improving women's health through advocacy, education, and research.

GHB
www.projectghb.org | Project GHB was started by Ken and Anya Shortridge after their son died from an overdose of GHB. Leading GHB and date rape drug expert Trinka Porrata has worked with the Shortridges to create this excellent resource for law enforcement as well as the public in date rape drug prevention and education.

Rape Treatment
www.911rape.org | This is the Web site for the UCLA Rape Treatment Center, one of the oldest and most experienced in the country. There are several rape treatment organizations available across the country. Of the numerous other long-standing organizations in the field, two of great reputation are the Rape, Abuse, and Incest National Network (www.rainn .org) and the Trauma Recovery Center (www .traumarecoverycenter.org).

www.ncvc.org | For information on the published paper from the National Center for Victims of Crime, "Rape in America; Report to the Nation."

CHAPTER 6: Facebook = Open Book
Cyberbullying
www.connectsafely.org | This is a forum designed to give teens and parents a voice in the public discussion about youth online safety.

www.opencongress.org/bill/110-h6123/ show | For help with cyberbullying and more information on the Megan Meier Cyberbullying Prevention Act. For Megan's story see www .meganmeierfoundation.org/story.

www.reclaimprivacy.org | This is an innovative open tool for scanning your Facebook privacy settings.

www.yoursphere.com | This site is a vibrant, interactive experience for kids and teens. As a member, you can safely surf and socialize online. Privacy comes first through common-sense safeguards that they have put in place.

ID Vault
www.idvault.com | ID Vault is a small device that plugs into a USB port and provides protection against identity theft and fraud for your online accounts. It encrypts your passwords, usernames, and credit card information; it logs you in without typing; and it creates a secure end-to-end connection between your computer and online accounts.

Online Harassment
www.haltabuse.org | Works to fight online harassment through education.

Sexting
www.sextingisstupid.org | A great Web site addressing the ramifications of sexting.

CHAPTER 7: ROAD TRIP!

Automobile Travel Support
www.aaa.com | The American Automobile Association represents the interests of motorists and other travelers. It is an invaluable resource for road safety.

Medical Concerns While Traveling
www.iamat.org | For help with medical issues when abroad, refer to the International Association for Medical Assistance to Travellers.

Spring Break
www.springbreaktravel.com | Provides information about reliable student travel packages.

Study Abroad

www.educationdynamics.com | This site has information on study abroad programs.

www.travel.state.gov | Always check with the U.S. Department of State for any travel questions, consulate information, or cultural climate concerns.

CHAPTER 8: Beware of the Bling

Consumers' Union

www.consumersunion.org | This site has credit card tips for college students.

Credit Counseling

www.nfcc.org | The National Foundation for Credit Counseling can help with credit card questions or with debt issues you might have.

Credit Protection

www.freecreditreport.com | A great service that monitors all your credit reports.

www.ftc.gov | For general credit card information on anything pertaining to fraud, contact the Federal Trade Commission.

www.ftc.gov/os/statutes/031224fcra.pdf | As a public service, the staff of the Federal Trade Commission (FTC) has prepared the complete text of the Fair Credit Reporting Act (FCRA), 15 U.S.C. § 1681 et seq.

www.lifelock.com | Lifelock is a service that not only monitors your bank and credit reports, but also guards other personal information such as your name, address, and Social Security number to alert you if someone is attempting to use your information for identity theft.

Identity Theft

www.fightidentitytheft.com | If you have been a victim of identity theft or want more information on the subject, visit the experts here.

CHAPTER 9: Stop—Don't Touch Me There!

www.ncadv.org | The National Coalition Against Domestic Violence organizes collective power by advancing transformative work, thinking, and leadership of communities and individuals working to end violence.

Sexual Harassment

www.eeoc.gov | The U.S. Equal Employment Opportunity Commission provides information about sexual harassment and you can file a formal charge through this site.

www.ovw.usdoj.gov/overview.htm | The Office on Violence against Women (OVW), a component of the U.S. Department of Justice, provides financial and technical assistance to communities across the country that are developing programs aimed at ending violence against women.

www.wrei.org | The Women's Research and Education Institute is an information and political analysis organization on women's equity.

CHAPTER 10: I'll Follow You Until You Love Me

Stalking

The following organizations can help with any stalking issue you might have. All of them are extremely comprehensive and are staffed with experienced people who can help.

www.feelsafeagain.org | A wonderful grass-roots nonprofit organization dedicated to helping stalking victims, especially on the East Coast.

www.lovemenot.org | Los Angeles District Attorney's Anti-Stalking Web site.

www.ncvc.org | 1-800-FYI-CALL | National Center for Victims of Crime (NCVC)

www.try-nova.org | National Association for Victim Assistance (NOVA).

Address Confidentiality Program (ACP)

www.ncadv.org/ | Visit this Website to find information on the program in your state.

U.S. Congressman Ed Royce

To read about U.S. Congressman Ed Royce and his legislation, go to **www.royce.house.gov**.

CHAPTER 11: Bring It On!

www.girlsfightback.com | For more information on Erin Weed and her company Girls Fight Back.

www.modelmugging.org | For more information on Matt Thomas and his organization Model Mugging.

www.taser.com | For information on the civilian TASER C2.

Spitfire Pepper Spray can be found at many retail locations, or go to **www.spitfire.us**.

A Sample Roommate Agreement (see Chapter 3, page 36, for more information on living with roommates)

This sample contract from Virginia Tech is a combined effort of several institutions and individuals, and is the ideal model for creating a useful agreement between you and your roommates.

You should contact your Student Legal Services on campus if you have any questions or need help with a lease or other legal issues. And you should see a licensed attorney for any legal advice or questions about landlord-tenant law.

ROOMMATE AGREEMENT

Reprinted with the permission of Virginia Tech University.
This Roommate Agreement is a legal and binding contract between the following Roommates:

1. Name: _____ SSN: _____

   Permanent Address: _____

2. Name: _____ SSN: _____

   Permanent Address: _____

3. Name: _____ SSN: _____

   Permanent Address: _____

4. Name: _____ SSN: _____

   Permanent Address: _____

1. Purpose of this Agreement. The purpose of this Agreement is to define the rights and obligations between the Roommates named above while living at

_____

_____

2. Choice of Law and Forum. This Agreement shall be governed by the laws of the Commonwealth of Virginia. All legal actions brought to enforce this contract shall be brought in the courts of Montgomery County, Virginia.

3. Incorporation of the Lease. All Roommates shall comply with the Lease. Any breach of the Lease by a Roommate is also a breach of this Roommate Agreement. Where there is a conflict between this Agreement and the Lease, the terms of the Lease shall have precedence.

4. Rent. Each Roommate shall pay his or her share of the rent as follows:

_____	$ _____ . ____
_____	$ _____ . ____
_____	$ _____ . ____
_____	$ _____ . ____

If the total amount of rent due under the lease changes, the change in rent shall be apportioned among the Roommates in proportion to the amount of rent shown above.

• •

Option A. If the lease requires payment of rent by a single check or money order for the entire unit, use this option.

_____ shall collect the rent from the other Roommates and make a single payment to the landlord (or its agent) pursuant to the terms of the lease. This Roommate is hereinafter referred to as the "Rent Payor" or "RP."

Each Roommate shall deliver to the RP full payment of his share of the rent by personal check, certified check, cashier's check, money order, or cash at least _____ days before the rent is due. The RP shall provide a receipt to any Roommate that requests one. Upon any Roommate's second late payment of rent resulting in damages, his rent shall be accelerated and he shall immediately pay the full amount of rent for the remainder of the lease term.

The RP shall pay in a manner that will provide him with proof of payment such as a receipt, a cancelled personal check, a debit on a bank account statement, or a credit card statement. To be valid, the proof of payment shall indicate the name of the payee, the amount paid, and the date the payment was deposited or debited. The RP shall save these receipts until one of the following events occurs: (1) the landlord returns the security deposit without deduction or claim for any rent owed, (2) a settlement regarding unpaid rent is made between the landlord and all of the Roommates, or (3) a claim for unpaid rent is resolved in court. The RP shall provide proof of payment to any Roommate upon request.

If, due to any fault of the RP, rent is not paid on time or receipts are not provided as requested, the other Roommates may elect to designate another person to be the RP. In such an event, the other Roommates shall provide the out-going RP written notice of his removal and the name of his replacement.

OR

*Option B. If the lease allows each Roommate to pay his rent separately,
use this option.*

Each Roommate shall pay his rent on time and shall pay in a manner that will provide
him with proof of payment such as a receipt, a cancelled personal check, a debit on a bank
account statement, or a credit card statement. To be valid, the proof of payment shall indicate
the name of the payee, the amount paid, and the date the payment was deposited or debited.
Each Roommate shall save these receipts until one of the following events occurs: (1) the
landlord returns the security deposit without deduction or claim for any rent owed, (2) a
settlement regarding unpaid rent is made between the landlord and all of the Roommates,
or (3) a claim for unpaid rent is resolved in court. If the landlord claims that rent is late,
Roommates shall provide proof of payment to any other Roommate upon request.

Each Roommate is liable for any damages resulting from a failure to pay rent or failure to
provide proof of payment and shall indemnify the other Roommates for any damages they
sustain due to his breach of this Agreement. Damages include, but aren't limited to, late
fees, interest, the landlord's attorney fees, and court costs. If the Roommates are evicted,
damages also include the moving expenses of the non-breaching Roommates and their
costs of a new tenancy, including rent for the remainder of the lease period.

Even if a Roommate vacates the premises, he shall continue to pay his full rent until the
lease expires or he is released in writing by all of the other Roommates.

5. Utilities. The Roommates agree to pay those utilities not included in the rent
according to the following amounts or shares:

Roommates

1	2	3	4

Payors

Local Phone Service:	LD Phone Service:	Cable Television:
Internet Service:	Electricity:	Gas:
Water:	Sewer:	Trash Pickup:
Lawn Service:		

The Roommates listed above as Payors shall have the indicated utilities placed in their
names. Each Payor shall collect the proper share of the utility charge from each Roommate
who is responsible for a share of the bill and make a single payment to the utility company
for which he is listed. At least ten days before a bill is due, the Payor shall notify the other
responsible Roommates of the amount of the bill and its due date. Those Roommates shall
pay the Payor their share of the bill at least five days before the bill is due. The Payor shall
provide a receipt to any Roommate that requests one.

The Payor shall provide access to the bills upon request of any Roommate. Roommates
who have not been provided with access to the bills upon reasonable request shall not be
responsible for any damages due to late payment of their share of this utility.

The Payor shall pay in a manner that will provide him with proof of payment such as a receipt, a cancelled personal check, a debit on a bank account statement, or a credit card statement. The proof of payment must indicate the name of the payee, the amount paid, and the date the payment was deposited or debited. The Payor shall provide proof of payment to any Roommate upon request. Damages resulting from failure to collect and save proof of payment shall be the full responsibility of the Payor.

If, due to any fault of the Payor, a utility bill is not paid on time or receipts are not provided as requested, the other Roommates may elect to designate another person to be the Payor. In such an event, the other Roommates shall provide the out-going Payor written notice of his removal and the name of his replacement.

Each Roommate is liable for any damages resulting from a failure to pay utilities or failure to provide proof of payment and shall indemnify the other Roommates for any damages they sustain due to his breach of this Agreement. Damages include, but aren't limited to, late fees, interest, reconnection fees, damages caused to persons or property from lack of heat, and diminishment of the value of the premises for the time period in which the utility was not available.

Even if a Roommate vacates the premises, he shall continue to pay his share of the utilities until the lease expires or he is released in writing by the other Roommates. If a vacating Roommate is a Payor, the remaining Roommates shall elect a new Payor and notify the outgoing Payor in writing.

6. Bounced Checks. If a Roommate pays by regular check and the check is drawn on insufficient funds (i.e., it "bounces"), that Roommate shall be responsible for all damages that result from this bounced check including, but not limited to, late fees and returned-check fees.

7. Property Damages. If the landlord requires submittal of a move-in inspection report, the first Roommate to move in shall complete and submit the report as required by the landlord and shall provide copies of the submitted report to the other Roommates.

If the landlord doesn't require submittal of a move-in inspection report, the first Roommate to move in shall draft a letter to the landlord (or its agent) listing all pre-existing damages. As each Roommate moves in, he shall inform the first Roommate of any damages that need to be listed, within three days of moving in. The first Roommate shall incorporate these additions into his letter, have each Roommate sign the letter, and submit the letter, within five days of the last Roommate's move-in, to the landlord (or its agent) by certified mail or hand delivery, in which case a hand receipt must be obtained. He shall also provide copies of the letter to the other Roommates.

Each Roommate shall pay for all damages he or his guests cause to the premises or to the personal property of any Roommate or guest. Any damages that cannot be traced to any particular party with reasonable certainty shall be paid equally by all Roommates. In the event of a dispute regarding responsibility for damages, the Roommates shall first try to negotiate the matter in good faith and then seek the help of a mediator or other neutral party mutually chosen by all Roommates before taking the matter to court.

8. Cleaning. All Roommates shall follow reasonable standards of cleanliness in maintaining the private and common areas of the premises. Roommates shall promptly address any concerns about cleanliness with each other in a polite and professional manner. Repeated requests to address any particular situation should be made in writing to the offending Roommate, and that Roommate shall sign for receipt of the written notice of these concerns.

If any Roommate's private room is kept in a fashion that attracts vermin (cockroaches, rats, etc.), the other Roommates may elect to provide the offending Roommate with written notice requiring him to remedy the condition within ten days of his receipt of the notice. If, despite being given proper notice, the offending Roommate fails to fix the condition in the required time, he shall be in breach of this contract. In such a case, the other Roommates may hire exterminators and cleaning-service providers to correct the problem and require the offender to pay the bill for any services rendered.

The Roommates shall abide by the following cleaning schedules and standards:

A. Kitchen
    Dishes: Sink: Refrigerator:
    Range: Microwave: Floors:
    Countertops:

B. Bathroom
    Toilet: Sink: Floor:
    Tub/Shower:

C. Trash Removal Schedule
D. Living Room, Dining Room, Den, and Hallways
E. Yard Work

9. Guests. The Roommates shall follow the lease and any rules and regulations indicated by the landlord governing guests. Except in case of an emergency, no Roommate shall invite or allow a guest to stay overnight or later than 11 p.m. if any Roommate will be attending classes or exams on the following day. No Roommate shall invite or allow a guest to spend the night on more than ___ occasions during any semester. Any Roommate who violates any provision in this paragraph without the express written permission of the other Roommates shall be liable to each Roommate for liquidated damages in the amount of $10.00 for each occurrence. Multiple guests count as multiple occurrences.

10. Parties and Gatherings. Roommates shall follow all lease terms, landlord rules and regulations, and local ordinances regarding parties, gatherings, noise, litter, and parking. No Roommate shall hold a party or gathering with more than three guests without the written consent of all of the other Roommates at least three days prior to the event. Consent shall not be unreasonably withheld. No Roommate shall hold a party in excess of twenty people, including Roommates, under any circumstances.

Any Roommate hosting a gathering or party shall, upon request of any other Roommate, terminate the event immediately.

All Roommates in attendance at a gathering or party shall share equally in cleaning the dwelling and removing trash and litter. They shall thoroughly clean the premises, deposit all trash in appropriate waste and recycling containers, and remove all litter left outside the dwelling by noon the following day. If the dwelling is an apartment, condo, or townhouse, outside litter shall be removed within one hour of the ending of the event but in no case any later than 7 a.m. the following morning.

11. Smoking. {Roommates may smoke inside the dwelling and permit their guests to do so as well.} OR {Roommates shall not smoke nor allow their guests to smoke inside the dwelling. A breach of this provision shall be deemed to have caused liquidated damages in the amount of $10.00 per each cigarette or cigar smoked payable to each non-offending Roommate.}

If smoking causes a fire on the property, the Roommate responsible for the fire shall pay for all damages caused by fire, smoke, or firefighting operations including, but not limited to, replacement of lost personal property, repairs to the dwelling, necessary moving expenses of any Roommate, and the cost of necessary replacement housing for a Roommate for the remainder of the original lease term.

12. Waiver. Waiver by any Roommate of any term or condition of this Agreement on any one occasion shall not waive the right to enforce that term or condition on any subsequent occasion.

13. Abandoned Property. If a Roommate vacates the premises for any reason and fails to remove his property within ten days, the property may be considered abandoned by the remaining Roommates. The remaining Roommates may sell or auction the abandoned property to satisfy any of the vacating Roommate's outstanding debts under this contract. If the vacating Roommate has no such debts, the remaining Roommates may divide the property amongst themselves as they see fit.

14. Forwarding Address and Phone Number. Each Roommate shall provide a forwarding address to each of the other Roommates at least ten days prior to vacating the premises for any reason (including termination of the lease). Each Roommate shall inform the other Roommates of any changes in his forwarding address within ten days of the change unless either the shares of the security deposit are returned in full to each Roommate or any disputes regarding damages are resolved by settlement or legal action. If any Roommate is compelled to use professional services to locate another Roommate's address for service of legal process, then the Roommate who failed to provide his forwarding address shall pay for the cost of determining his location.

15. General Courtesy. Each Roommate shall be reasonable and professional in his dealings with the other Roommates and refrain from any behavior, action, or inaction that he knows or has reason to believe will significantly interfere with another Roommate's enjoyment of the tenancy. Each Roommate agrees to negotiate in good faith, should the need arise. Each Roommate shall respect the other Roommates' privacy, sleep schedules, and reasonable requests.

16. Criminal Behavior. Roommates shall not commit any crime on the premises that either (1) interferes with the rights of another Roommate (including, but not limited to, larceny, damage to property, assault, battery, fraud, invasion of privacy, harassment, and stalking), (2) involves inherently dangerous activities, violent acts, or weapon violations, or (3) jeopardizes the continued right of the other Roommates to occupy the premises under the terms of the lease. Such activity shall be a breach of this agreement.

Any Roommate convicted of one of the crimes listed above shall immediately vacate the premises, regardless of the status of any appeal. The convicted tenant shall remain responsible for his portion of the rent and utilities as defined elsewhere in this agreement.

17. Firearms and Other Weapons. Roommates {may} OR {shall not} keep firearms, bows, hunting or combat knives, machetes, or other weapons on the premises.

Weapons shall be stored in the following manner(s):

_____

Any Roommate keeping a weapon on the premises in violation of this section shall be liable to each of the other Roommates for liquidated damages in the amount of $50.00 per violation.

18. Resolution of Disputes. All Roommates shall resolve their disputes in a fair and mature fashion and shall seek the help of a mediator or alternative dispute resolution agency if they are unable to agree on their own. All Roommates shall share the cost of any mediation or alternative dispute resolution. The results of any negotiation or mediation shall be recorded or reduced to writing for the review of all Roommates.

If it is necessary to litigate any dispute arising under this Agreement, the losing Roommate shall pay all court costs, reasonable collection costs, and reasonable attorney fees.

19. Signatures. We, the undersigned, hereby indicate by our signatures below that we have read this full agreement, that we understand all it contains, that we agree to be bound by its terms and conditions, and that it is the complete statement of our understanding of the terms and conditions of our tenancy together.

_____

Signature | Date

_____

Signature | Date

_____

Signature | Date

_____

Signature | Date

The Safety Chick Stalking Incident Log

You can make copies of this form and use it for your records.

Your name: _____ Your contact number: _____

Description of Suspect

Name: _____ Sex: ____

Race: _____

Date of birth: _____

Height and weight: _____ pounds, _____

Eye color : _____ Hair color: _____

Home address: _____

Home or cell phone number: _____

Work address: _____

Work phone number: _____

Vehicle description (make, model, color, license plate number): _____

INCIDENT REPORT

Date: _____ Time: _____

Location: _____

Description of incident/evidence collected: _____

_____

_____

_____

Names and phone numbers of witnesses: _____

_____

_____

_____

Police report #: _____ Name/badge # of reporting officer: _____

Index

Acknowledgments

To all the experts in this book who contributed their invaluable information and expertise—thank you for dedicating your lives to helping victims and keeping people safe from crime: Bernice Sandler, Trinka Porata, UC Davis Police Chief Annette Spicuzza, University of Wisconsin—Madison Police Chief Susan Riseling, Tom Quilty, Mary Kay Hoal, Matt Thomas, Julio Mercado, and Kathryn (Keith) Sims.

To my family:

Dad and Mom: You are always loyal, loving, and go above and beyond to help me succeed. My brothers Kevin and Rob: Thanks for making me tough. My three boys, Turner, Landon, and Ramsey: Thanks for making me even tougher—and reminding me *every day* the importance of living with strength, courage, and common sense—I am proud and honored to be your Momma.

To my friends and colleagues:

Ron Brooks: Again, you will always be my lifesaver. You are one heck of a cop. United States Congressman Ed Royce: For changing my life and that of victims everywhere. My editor Laura Lee Mattingly: You definitely earned your "Safety Chick Stripes"! Thanks for your help making this book exceptional.

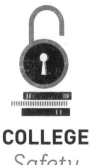

COLLEGE
Safety
101